The Human Drama of Abortion

A Global Search for Consensus

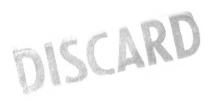

The Human Drama of Abortion
A Global Search for Consensus

Aníbal Faúndes

José Barzelatto

Vanderbilt University Press
Nashville

© 2006 Vanderbilt University Press
All rights reserved
First Edition 2006

10 09 08 07   2 3 4 5

Printed on acid-free paper.
Manufactured in the United States of America

Library of Congress Cataloging-in-Publication Data

Faúndes, Aníbal, 1931–
[Drama do Aborto. English]
The human drama of abortion : seeking a global consensus / Aníbal
Faúndes, José Barzelatto.— 1st ed.
     p. ; cm.
Includes bibliographical references and index.
ISBN 0-8265-1525-8 (cloth : alk. paper)
ISBN 0-8265-1526-6 (pbk. : alk. paper)
     1. Abortion—Cross-cultural studies. 2. Pregnancy, Unwanted—
Cross-cultural studies. [DNLM: 1. Abortion, Induced. 2. Family
Planning Services. 3. Health Policy. 4. Pregnancy, Unwanted.
5. Women's Rights. HQ 767 F258d 2006a]
I. Barzelatto, J. (José) II. Title.
     HQ767.F38 2006
     363.46—dc22   2005028168

To Ellen and Juanita, our lifetime companions,
who helped us understand what it means
to be a woman in today's world.

Contents

Part II: Values

Part III: Improving the Situation

Part IV: Seeking a Consensus

Acknowledgments

We begin by acknowledging the unexpected and profound influence of our joint residency at the Rockefeller Foundation's Bellagio Study and Conference Center, where we arrived with only an agreed-upon book outline and a very rough draft of some sections. The atmosphere at the center and the people we met there helped us in a number of ways. First, although we had been friends for decades, the environment permitted us to get to know each other even better. This proved to be essential, both during and after our stay at Bellagio, because it allowed us to maintain a respectful and constructive dialogue during the many instances in which we found we had minor but significant differences in perspective. Second, the people we met at Bellagio, many of whom were very interested in the subject matter of this text and were willing to discuss their personal views, influenced the way we structured the book. In particular, we thank Lou Stein, who took the time to read some of the early drafts and made valuable editorial suggestions, and Ruth Macklin, whose profound knowledge of bioethics provided many important insights.

We also thank the friends and colleagues who read initial drafts for their invaluable support and suggestions, which reflected not only their vast experience but also their great wisdom: Frank Alvarez, Vivian Brache, Horacio Croxatto, Elizabeth Dawson, Raul Faúndes, Christine Gudorf, Ellen Hardy, and Stephen Isaacs.

In addition, we are grateful to Susan Godstone and Lesley Hanson de Moura for their editorial assistance. Susan began by correcting our grammatical errors and improving our English usage. Then Lesley greatly enhanced the style and offered excellent suggestions with respect to the content. We also acknowledge the dedicated and competent technical support of Cecilia Barros, who coordinated the many versions of both text and references that traveled back and forth through cyberspace for more than two years.

Finally, we express our appreciation for the contribution of the many women who, over the past fifty years of our professional lives, have shared their experiences with us, confided their stories to us, and conveyed to us in their own words what abortion really means to them. We dedicate this book to all of these women, without whom it could not have been written.

First Preface

As I was working on this book, I realized how much of my life has been dedicated to dealing with the human drama of abortion. Neither biography nor memoir, this book clearly has its origin in the emotional impact of the suffering of women with abortion complications that I experienced as a young intern at a public hospital in Santiago de Chile in 1953. Witnessing the physical and psychological pain of both younger and older women for weeks on end, listening to their stories, and watching them either die or survive in a severely mutilated state was a strong motivation for me to dedicate a large part of my professional life to finding a way to mitigate their suffering.

For many years I believed that family planning alone was the answer, and I took on the unusual role for an obstetrician (rather than a gynecologist) of working in many different countries in various areas of contraception, from the development of new contraceptive methods to the planning and implementation of nationwide family planning programs. Only after decades of working in the field did it become clear to me that family planning alone was not a sufficient response. I learned that other social initiatives were of equal importance in reducing the number of women who saw abortion as the only way out: the promotion of a fair gender power balance, the availability of sex education for both male and female adolescents, and protection against family and societal rejection for women who choose to keep their babies.

In addition to my belief in the necessity of helping women avoid unwanted pregnancy, I was moved by the social injustice of penalizing women who abort. It is impossible to hear their stories without concluding that these women, far from being criminals, are victims of the ways in which societies are organized. Their biggest sin is being poor, because even in countries where abortion is legally restricted, women of means can obtain clean, safe abortions.

My heartfelt need to help reduce the suffering caused by unwanted pregnancy and by the criminalization of abortion awakened my realization that the global majority has an incomplete view of the issue and that this widespread dearth of information is the main obstacle to achieving an understanding of and a solution to the problem.

This book, therefore, has the rather utopian intention of influencing politicians and policymakers to adopt and implement social initiatives that have proven effective in reducing abortion and minimizing its consequences on women and on society. Because politicians are moved by public opinion, however, this book has also been written with the hope of reaching a broader audience who will help influence those who have the power to implement social change.

—Aníbal Faúndes

Second Preface

As a student and then as a young physician at a university hospital in Chile from the late 1940s to the 1960s, I witnessed the growing epidemic and national tragedy of women who suffered the complications of unsafe abortions, and I was emotionally marked by the experience forever. Although at that time my field of work was internal medicine and I did not have the obstetrical experience of my coauthor, I cared for many women whose late complications following a botched abortion commonly resulted in death. Like most of my colleagues, I was also appalled at the number of women who came to our hospitals to give birth, only to be hurried home within twenty-four hours of delivery after being forced to share a hospital bed with another woman, in order to free beds for the increasing number of women who suffered abortion complications.

At the time, Chile was in the process of becoming industrialized, and low-income women had finally begun to gain access to work in the factories, allowing them to contribute to family income and help increase family status. This new status for women demanded a smaller-family norm, which was facilitated by a progressive drop in child mortality. Women no longer needed to have many children in order to have a few that would survive. In the absence of effective modern contraceptives, the number of abortions increased dramatically, despite the fact that they were legally restricted. The outrage of the Chilean medical profession brought about a government response, which made modern contraceptives freely and widely available through the nation's National Health Service.

Aware that they had been risking their lives, women who had resorted to abortion began using contraceptives as soon as they became available. The results were spectacular. The number of women hospitalized for complications from unsafe abortions, which had been growing steadily over the previous twenty years, decreased by 50 percent within five years and continued to decrease in subsequent years, as deaths from abortion dropped to one-sixth of their previous level. Within a few short years, the dramatic fall in the number of beds occupied by women with abortion complications meant that the days of two women sharing one maternity ward bed were over.

Chilean society at large and the majority of the country's health professionals were satisfied with the good, albeit partial, results brought about by the accessibility of modern contraceptives, and they pursued the problem of unsafe abortion no further. Abortion was still considered immoral, a sin; legal restriction therefore continued. The tragic consequences for low-income women were ignored. Consequently, unnecessary suffering and death resulting from illegal abortion, although decreased in magnitude, remain a significant social and public health problem to this day.

Since the mid-1960s, my international professional experience has taught me the following: (1) abortion is a global problem, (2) despite characteristics peculiar to different societies, some basic issues are shared, and (3) the number of abortions can be reduced everywhere if we can clarify misunderstandings and thus convert current conflicts into a practical political consensus that will allow the implementation of effective policies.

It is the intention of this book to offer, in a single volume for nonspecialists, the lessons of our experience, both national and international, including all important factors that we have learned about abortion. Our aim is to provide information for public and political discussion, in an effort to enlighten a public debate that has been characterized by extremism and impassioned argument. Both intellectual integrity and mutual respect are needed to fuel a constructive debate.

—José Barzelatto

Introduction

Many excellent works on abortion have been published in recent years. Why go to the trouble and effort of writing another book on the subject? We felt an urgent need to do so because we believe that the thousands of pages published in books, in scientific journals, and in the lay press on the subject of abortion do not provide an easily readable, comprehensive view of the issue. We are convinced that providing more factual information is crucial to a better understanding of this personal and social problem, which affects most people directly or indirectly sometime in their lives. Even more important, it is clear to us that without this understanding it will be almost impossible to find a solution to this problem that has such profound physical and emotional implications for so many people in the world today.

Most books published on the subject of abortion concentrate on one aspect of the problem and address an audience already involved in the philosophical, religious, social, or health aspects of the debate. Because these books are not geared toward the general public, most people do not read them and consequently, do not take an active role in the public discussion. This book was written to be accessible to anyone interested in abortion, because we believe this is a subject that affects virtually everyone. There is a need for current and comprehensive information that can help dissipate the prevailing misunderstandings surrounding abortion. We believe that once the "silent" majority is better informed, the cultural changes required in order to reach a political consensus will become possible.

In addition, an accessible and comprehensive review of the abortion issue is essential for nonspecialized opinion leaders and policymakers, who receive most of their information from the opposing views of an excessively polarized public debate dominated by ideological emotions. It is our view that this situation could be greatly improved if both policymakers and the general public would recognize the false dilemma of having to be either for or against abortion.

Why do we even attempt to take on the enormous task at hand? As our prefaces indicate, we are two physicians from a developing country, both with broad international experience, who have been involved in the problem of abortion since we attended medical school. We have both lived for decades outside our country of birth but remain deeply involved in the human drama of abortion in many different ways and in many different countries around the world. This book reflects what we have learned by personal experience throughout our lives.

Abortion is a word that elicits profound emotions in all of us, irrespective of our level of involvement with the issue or the degree of concern shown by the societies in which we live. The twentieth century witnessed a heated rhetorical confrontation between two extreme positions, each of which appeared incapable of taking the other into account or of maintaining a civilized and rational discussion. We postulate that those who adopt such extreme positions, although they claim to represent a large group, actually constitute a relatively small minority. In reality, most people's position with respect to abortion, far from being radical, falls somewhere within a broad range of opinions. Because this less radical majority does not broach the issue with the passion of the extremists, it is less vocal in public. As a result, past and (to an even greater degree) recent public discussions on abortion have been dominated by the two radical extremes.

At one extreme are those who believe that the embryo or fetus must take absolute priority over women's personal decisions and who seem to completely ignore the rights of women. At the other extreme are those who give absolute priority to women's right to decide for themselves whether to continue or terminate a pregnancy and seem to ignore any possible value of the embryo or fetus. These two extremes are represented in the pro-life and pro-choice movements, respectively. Radical pro-life activists consider only the fetus's right to life, disregarding not only the circumstances and quality of the woman's life and the lives of her other children but also the baby's own future. Pro-choice radicals, in turn, negate all value of the embryo or fetus. Neither extreme is open to respectful consideration of the arguments of the other. Any indication that one is willing to pay attention to the arguments of the other is seen as a sign of weakness of conviction, an inroad for the "enemy's" argument. The controversy is so heated and the emotions are so strong that polarization of public opinion has become very difficult to avoid. It is our argument that this is a false dilemma—that the great majority of people in the world are not indifferent to the suffering of the millions of women who confront the decision to abort every year. The same majority is also not indifferent to the fate of the fetus and sees every abortion as a loss.

The idea that people are divided between those for and those against abortion is simply incorrect. It is, in fact, a great misunderstanding of the real issue. In our experience, the vast majority of both factions is against abortion *per se*. In other words, most people believe that a world without abortion would be a better place for all—but at the same time the vast majority accepts the idea that, under certain circumstances, an induced abortion can be an acceptable moral choice.

If the opposing sides realized the lesser degree of their differences, we believe it would open the door to a constructive dialogue that could lead to a consensus on at least some vital points. It is our contention that once a rational, civilized dialogue is begun, almost everyone— including the less radical of the two extremes —will agree to the promotion and implementation of the social changes that have proven to reduce the incidence and the consequences of induced abortion. We believe that this is a difficult but not an impossible task. The aim of this book is to help initiate such a dialogue.

In addition, this book is of interest not only to students, teachers, and activists involved in human rights issues in general and sexual and reproductive rights in particular but also to those who deal with sex education, family life and religion, and public health problems. This includes societies the world over, because the controversy of abortion is universal.

Throughout this book, we illustrate our points using real-life stories that we have witnessed in various countries. Each situation evolved as described; however, except where we were authorized to relate the stories intact, we have changed names and extraneous details to respect the privacy of those involved. We thank everyone whose story gave us and will, we hope, give our readers, a better understanding of the human drama of abortion.

This book is divided into four parts:

Part I: The Human Drama of Abortion describes the main aspects of the complex personal and social problem of abortion. We start by listening to women explain why they decided to have an abortion and then clarify the meanings of the terms used in relation to the issue. A worldwide review of the problem—its alarming magnitude and its tragic consequences—follows. The section ends with an analysis of why women get pregnant when they do not want to and when pregnancy becomes so unwanted that women decide to abort.

Part II: The Values Involved starts by describing the conflicting values faced by health professionals who deal with abortions. It goes on to review the religious and ethical values that influence the behavior of all those involved and ends with an overview of the reflection of these values in the legislation of countries around the world.

Part III: Improving the Situation, while taking into account the facts stated in Part I and the values discussed in Part II, reviews the interventions that have proven effective in decreasing the number of abortions and in reducing the human, social, and economic costs. The section ends by describing the paradoxical position of groups that perceive their role as staunch campaigners in the fight against abortion but that remain opposed to many of the interventions which have proven to be effective means of abortion reduction.

Part IV: Seeking a Consensus closes the book by analyzing the need for societies to reach a political agreement about abortion. It is our belief that this is an achievable task because it is possible for reasonable people with very different overall views to identify and expand common ideas and shared values that can become the basis for a political consensus. To this end, and based on the evidence described in the first three parts of the book, Part IV identifies nine such significant points and consequent actions that might provide the basis for a social consensus that would allow societies to deal more effectively with the human drama of abortion. The book ends with a commentary on the process required to reach this goal, which is the final aim of this book.

PART I

The Human Drama
of Abortion

1
Listening to Women
Why They Have Abortions

Only women know exactly why they end up making the difficult decision to have an abortion. Consequently, there is no better way to help us understand the issue than to listen to their stories. The story of each woman, rich or poor, younger or older, illiterate or highly educated—related here as told to us over the years—is unique and serves to illustrate the variety of circumstances that lead women to choose to terminate their pregnancies.

The Story of a Peasant

Rosa belonged to a family of peasants, and her husband worked a small piece of land. She had had six children, one after the other, with the interval between them determined only by prolonged breastfeeding. One had died of diarrhea before his second birthday. Rosa looked old and wasted for her thirty-one years. She was always the first to get up to prepare breakfast and to see that the children were ready in time to go to school. She did not want them to have to go through the same hard, painful experience that she had gone through on so many occasions when there was not always enough food, particularly during the two years of drought, when even the cow had almost died of starvation.

The older child, a twelve-year-old boy, was his father's pride, but he was of no help to his mother. It was her ten-year-old daughter, who often stepped in and took care of her younger siblings. At this pont, it was clear to Rosa that five children were enough. God alone knew how difficult it was for her to keep them all well fed, dressed, clean, and loved. Her mother, however, said that children were a blessing that God gives to women and that Rosa should be grateful to receive them. Her mother's influence lost much of its strength after the birth of Rosa's seventh child.

As usual, Rosa gave birth at home. The placenta was retained, and she bled heavily. Luckily, the only neighbor who had a car was home and could rush her to the hospital in town. At the hospital, Rosa had to undergo a massive blood transfusion to save her life. Before she left the hospital, the doctor who had saved her explained that another pregancy could kill her and she should not have any more children. He forgot, however, to tell her what to do to avoid pregnancy. Rosa had heard about birth control pills but did not have the money to purchase them every month. Someone at church taught her how to use the rhythm method, but her husband would not always agree to abstain during her fertile days of the month, and she did not dare go against his wishes.

Rosa was terrified of the possibility of getting pregnant again and leaving six small children without a mother. She followed the advice of her mother and neighbors, using herbal vaginal douches after coitus, but eventually her menstruation was late again. She drank all kinds of herbal teas and took all kinds of medications she got at the pharmacy to no avail. Then she was told that all the herbal concoctions and drugs she had taken would have damaged the fetus, which would be severely deformed if the pregnancy were allowed to continue. Finally, she went to the local abortionist, who succeeded in causing uterine bleeding. The abortion was completed at a hospital, where she was taken with a severe infection from which she recovered after a few days. This time, determined not to take anymore chances, the doctor offered her a surgical sterilization, which she gratefully accepted.

A Middle-Class Urban Woman

Maria was a thirty-four-year-old married woman with four children. Her husband worked in a bank and earned a good salary. The family lived a comfortable life, but expenses increased as the children grew. Public education was inadequate, tuition at the private school they were attending had risen, and Maria and her husband wanted all their children to have the opportunity to go to college. The couple had intended to have only three children, but Maria had tired of using the pill and they had decided to stop for a few months and practice abstinence during the fertile period of the menstrual cycle.

The method had failed, and five years after the birth of her third child, Maria had given birth to her fourth child. A doctor had recommended the use of the copper IUD, but Maria was concerned about a neighbor's allegation that the IUD caused a small abortion every month. As a result, Maria decided to go back to the pill while she tried to obtain a surgical sterilization. During her summer vacation, however, she was three days late in starting a new cycle of pills. She was unaware of the risk involved in missing those few days of pills until her menses failed to appear When she failed to menstruate, she was in despair; she could not possibly have another baby. Maria had always rejected the idea of abortion and had even criticized women who resorted to abortion. Now, however, she could see no alternative; she had to protect the future of her four children.

Her husband agreed and was verbally supportive, but he did not know how to proceed. Maria went to see the doctor who had delivered all her babies. The doctor was as friendly as she had always known him to be, but he tried to dissuade her from her decision to have an abortion. She insisted, however, explaining that even her last child—God bless him—was putting an enormous burden on the family. They were struggling to provide a decent education for the four children they already had. With an additional child, it would be impossible to make ends meet. Her doctor understood Maria's dilemma, but he did not perform abortions, which were illegal in their country. After Maria pleaded for the doctor's assistance, explaining that she had no idea where to go for help, he gave her a piece of paper with a telephone number and address.

Maria called the number that same evening. The abortion would be quite expensive, but other than cost, there were no obstacles. Maria and her husband did not have the money on hand and the clinic that would perform the abortion accepted only cash, but she did not want to wait any longer. With great reluctance, she told the whole story to her mother. To Maria's surprise, her mother was was more supportive than she had ever imagined; only then did she learn that her mother had once gone through the same experience herself. Maria's mother not only gave her the money she needed but accompanied her to the clinic when her husband gave all kinds of excuses for not going with her. The abortion went smoothly, and Maria's mother's support greatly strengthened her emotional well-being.

A Young, Idealistic Career Woman

Blanca was the first-born child of a wealthy farmer who had only two daughters. Blanca's mother had died when she was six years old, and her father had kept her under a tight rein throughout her adolescence. She soon realized that the only way to become independent was to have her own career and earn her own money. Mindful of the fact that a medical error had caused the death of her mother, she decided to study medicine. Her acceptance into medical school had the additional advantage of allowing her to leave home and live independently in the big city. She was a good student and dedicated most of her free time to sports. Ever since her youth, she had spent hours running, seemingly tirelessly, up and down the hills. Now the university environment inspired her to run in competitions, which she always bested. Blanca had inherited from her mother a pretty face; lovely dark eyes; and long, thick ebony hair. With her slim body and winning smile, she had captured the attention of classmates and acquaintances, but she had never fallen deeply in love with any of her suitors. Obeying her father's strict moral rules of conduct, she had remained a virgin until just before she finished medical school.

For her year of medical practice, Blanca had chosen an extremely deprived and isolated spot. She was very sensitive to the suffering of the poor in her country and wanted to use her medical training to be of help. It was there that she met Guillermo, a young, handsome, charming leader of the peasant union, who shared her intense dedication to social justice. Admiration soon turned into love, and after a short and passionate courtship, they were married. Her father's resistance dissipated when he learned that she was already pregnant. She gave birth to a beautiful daughter, Camila, delivered at home with the help of a traditional birth attendant. Blanca wanted everything to be natural and did not want any privileges that the people around her did not have. Not everything in her life was perfect, however. Beginning in the final months of her pregnancy, her beloved husband had begun to pay less and less attention to her. The couple had continued to have sexual intercourse, but Blanca no longer felt any desire to make love. Blanca had begun to realize that she took second place to her husband's passion for the cause of the peasants, which consumed all his energy and attention. As they grew increasingly distant in the months following their daughter's birth, Blanca became acutely aware that their marriage had no future. She did not regret having married her husband and was very happy with her daughter, but that was the extent of it. She felt the need to resume her career, to help the people of her community, but she kept putting off a decision to separate from her husband.

As part of her determination to live a life close to nature, Blanca used no "artificial" contraception. She expected that breastfeeding would at least partially protect her from pregnancy, and she did her best to avoid sex during her fertile period, placing Camila between Guillermo and herself in their bed and using every excuse to reject his advances. However, when he insisted on claiming his spousal rights, she felt unable to refuse him and had sexual intercourse against her will. To her dismay, her efforts proved inadequate, and she became pregnant again. Blanca was in no doubt about what to do. Having already decided that her life with Guillermo had come to an end and that she had to be able to keep working to support Camila and herself, she knew that she could not go through another pregnancy and have another child. She knew exactly where to go, and before the end of her ninth week of pregnancy, she had an abortion. She then separated from Guillermo and started a new life fulfilled by Camila and her work. Blanca was sure that her decision to abort this pregnancy was as right for her as had been her decision to give birth to Camila.

A Mature, Well-to-Do Physician

Cristina was a thirty-eight-year-old physician happily married to a successful lawyer who was ten years her senior. The couple lived with their two preadolescent children. Their sex life had become monotonous and sporadic, and because Cristina did not like taking hormones, they used either a condom or a diaphragm as contraception. Because Cristina had required medical help to achieve both of her pregnancies, she doubted that she was still fertile.

The monotony of her marriage was broken when, during a medical convention, she had met Antonio, a foreign colleague a few years her junior, who had made her feel attractive again. She had welcomed a seemingly innocent flirtation and had very much enjoyed their conversations. She had never been unfaithful to her husband, for whom she felt an unwavering affection, and she valued the security of her family. She had never imagined that this "professional" relationship would go any further. Six months after she and Antonio had first met, however, she accepted an invitation to lecture at a medical seminar at a vacation resort in another country. Her husband had professional commitments during that period and was unable to accompany her. As she was checking in at the hotel, she ran into Antonio. They both felt an immediate attraction.

During the days that followed, Antonio managed to be around her almost constantly. He invited her for dinner, and she accepted. Romance was very much in the air. They danced and talked for hours and ended up making passionate love. Cristina was aware that she was close to her fertile period and was using no protection, but she felt completely helpless to resist this man who appeared to be so passionately in love with her.

Back home, she treasured her memories while at the same time she tried to forget what had happened. But when she failed to menstruate, she realized that she was pregnant. Fortunately, because of the infrequency of Cristina's sexual encounters with her husband, he paid little attention to her menstrual cycle and was unaware of any change. Cristina had no doubt that for the sake of her family and her future she could not allow the pregnancy to continue. She invented a visit to her mother, who lived in another city, and had a safe, and expensive, abortion. She felt an immense sense of relief, told no one about the episode, and promised herself that she would never make the same mistake again.

A Working-Class Teenager

The story of *Luisa* is very different. Luisa was eighteen years old, the oldest child in a lower-middle-class family of three children. Her father worked in a factory and earned a reasonably good living, not enough to keep his family in luxury but enough to maintain a small, two-room apartment in a government-sponsored compound. Luisa worked during the day as a sales clerk in an elegant boutique in the best shopping center in town. She was a nice-looking girl, tall and slim, and the owner had hired her for her appearance and her very warm and easy smile. Luisa had interrupted her studies to take the job the previous year, but she had now resumed school in the evenings after work.

It was in the boutique that she met Carlos, who was Christmas shopping with his mother. Although they had spoken only a few words, his soft, warm voice and his shy manner had captivated her.

Carlos came back the next day to purchase a small item and asked her to join him for some ice cream after work. Luisa accepted happily. Carlos, she learned, was a twenty-one-year-old university student, the only son in an affluent family, which provided him with a car and more money than Luisa had ever earned. They soon fell deeply in love, and and it was only a question of time until they would have sex. Luisa knew how to protect herself, and when it had become clear that sexual intercourse was inevitable, she had started to take the pill.

The relationship continued to intensify in the following months, but Carlos's reluctance to meet her parents was beginning to make her uneasy. When Luisa started to have severe, recurrent headaches, she made an appointment at the family planning clinic. The doctor gave her a diaphragm and told her that she had to stop taking the pill. Luisa complied, and the headaches disappeared. Three months later, she realized that her menstruation was late. She waited another two weeks and then went back to the clinic. A urine test confirmed that she was pregnant.

Luisa had conflicting feelings about this state of affairs. She was uneasy about the circumstances, but she was also happy to be expecting the child of the man she loved so dearly. She realized, in fact, that it was something she had subconsciously wanted. She would be able to continue working, she already had some savings, and if Carlos's family continued to provide him with his monthly allowance, Luisa and Carlos would be able to afford a reasonable lifestyle until he finished his studies and began his career. She realized that it would be impossible to continue her education after the baby was born, but that was a sacrifice she was willing to make. Carlos and the baby would be her life from then on.

The following Saturday Carlos came to pick her up after work, and they went directly to a motel. He was as tender and loving as ever and seemed anxious to be with her. When they were lying in each other's arms, after they had made love, she told him the news. Carlos appeared shocked. "Are you sure?" he asked. "How did this happen when you were taking the pill?" Luisa explained that she had had to stop taking the pill and that the diaphragm occasionally fails. To her surprise, for the first time in their relationship, Carlos was furious: How could she have done this to him? He had been so dedicated to her, had even abandoned his old friends for her, and now she had done this terrible thing to him. With great difficulty, Luisa explained her plans. Carlos looked at her as if he were seeing her for the first time. "Are you crazy?" he said. "Why are you doing this to me? If you want to stay with me, you'll have to get rid of this pregnancy right now!" Luisa could not believe her ears; she could do nothing but cry. Carlos's reaction could not have been more different from what she had expected! He tried to calm her down, to no avail, and they separated without another word about the pregnancy.

When Luisa's mother saw her daughter arrive at the family home, she immediately realized that something was very wrong. After some hesitation, Luisa told her everything. She said that she wanted to keep the child and that she expected her parents' support. Her mother did her best to discourage this decision and her father would not accept it—this would be the end of her dream of a career and a better life. Furthermore, Luisa's mother knew where she could get an abortion and would find the money to pay for it

Luisa did not want to take her mother's advice. She wanted to keep her baby. It was a part of her true love that she could keep forever, and perhaps Carlos would change his mind after their baby was born. She decided to ask her boss for help. The boutique owner was an open-minded woman who had supported Luisa's efforts to continue her studies at night. Once again, however, Luisa was greatly disappointed. The shop owner was understanding and supportive, but also made it perfectly clear that she did not want a pregnant woman working in her elegant boutique. Although, in theory, Luisa was legally protected from losing her job as a result of her pregnancy, her boss had the resources to get around the law. Luisa's job was her only means of economic support for the baby and herself. She resisted for awhile, but after a few days of continuous pressure from her mother and her boss, she had to agree to abort the pregnancy that she had wanted so much.

Real-life stories such as these abound. The stories described here are merely examples of situations that have led women to abort. The women in these stories are all from Latin America, and their circumstances may differ from those of women from other regions, cultures, and socioeconomic environments. Even in Latin America, there are numerous different stories to be told. The common ground, however, is that all of these women are faced with no alternative but to terminate their pregnancies. There is no doubt that women do not have abortions because they enjoy the experience. Every woman we have known who has had an abortion would have preferred to avoid it. Although most of them were satisfied with their decision to abort and had no regrets at having done so, they would have been much happier if the need had not arisen. Many other authors in developed and developing countries have documented the same experience (Bengtsson and Wahlberg, 1991; Kero et al., 1999; Alvarez et al., 1999; Kero and Lalos, 2000).

Clearly, abortion occurs because a pregnancy was unintended or later became unwanted. By analyzing why the women in the stories described here made the decision to abort, we are able to distinguish two different dimensions: the circumstances that led them to a pregnancy that they did not want and the reasons that giving birth to the child was not an option at that particular time. We will discuss each of these two aspects separately in Chapters 5 and 6 and will use the above stories as examples.

2
The Meaning of Words

I (JB) was visiting a Muslim country, representing the World Health Organization (WHO). Soon after my arrival, I received an unexpected invitation to meet with a high official of the Ministry of Health. I felt both obliged to accept and excited about the opportunity to acquire firsthand knowledge of the Ministry of Health's policies on reproductive health.

A few days later, the official received me, and we exchanged a few polite words. After he expressed his gratitude for the collaboration of WHO and I expressed my pleasure at the opportunity to visit his fascinating country, he immediately launched into a twenty-minute discourse on the evils of induced abortion. He expounded upon every negative aspect of terminating a normal pregnancy, including the effect it can have on health and the family; most emphatic, however, were his statements about the negative moral and religious implications of induced abortion. He left no doubt whatsoever about his complete opposition to abortion.

The speech took me totally by surprise, as my visit had nothing to do with abortion. As my host talked, I wondered why he focused so intently on explaining that his government would categorically reject any initiative to facilitate safe abortion. I wondered which of my planned activities had inspired this forceful statement. My curiosity was satisfied when we finally came to the point of our meeting: Would WHO, he asked, help his country expand a national program on menstrual regulation?

This request caught me completely off guard, since for me, as for most people, menstrual regulation is considered a form of early abortion. It was clear, however, that in order to make the request, it had been politically and religiously mandatory for my host to separate menstrual regulation from later abortion and it was equally clear that his government would never accept any similarity between the two procedures. My host was unaware of the important lesson he was giving me about how crucial it is to use the appropriate words when referring to abortion, in accordance with the context and the cultural, political and religious environment.

The Need to Define Terms Related to Abortion

Abortion is usually defined as the abnormal termination of pregnancy, spontaneous or induced. Spontaneous abortion, the termination of a pregnancy without any external intervention, can be caused by a disease in the pregnant woman or by genetic defects in the embryo. Induced abortion is the termination of a pregnancy by intentional external intervention.

Spontaneous abortion is basically a medical problem that affects a woman's health, although it may also involve social and psychological consequences for both the woman and her family. Induced abortion is both a personal and a social problem with profound medical, cultural, religious, ethical, political, and psychological implications. This book refers exclusively to the problems associated with induced abortions, and throughout it we will always use the word "abortion" to mean induced abortion.

Medical terms are usually defined by the WHO and then become generally accepted by most people involved in health care. In the case of pregnancy and abortion, however, a knowledge gap and political agendas have led to the existence of varied definitions, particularly when the confusion has helped manipulate the debate over abortion. The fact that a constructive exchange of ideas requires an agreement on the meaning of key words is frequently overlooked. A lack of agreement on meaning has been a basic flaw in the ongoing global abortion debate in recent decades. The use of agreed-upon definitions or awareness of and clarification of the use of different definitions are crucial to the prevention of misunderstandings.

Medical definitions of pregnancy and abortion are based on the biological body of knowledge about human reproduction. To fully understand these definitions, we must first review what is currently known about the reproductive process.

The Reproductive Process

It is common knowledge that following sexual intercourse a woman sometimes becomes pregnant and that when she does, in most cases nine months later a new individual is born. Since sex is not always followed by pregnancy, however, how do we know when pregnancy has started and when, therefore, either a spontaneous or an induced abortion is possible? When menstruation is delayed, a woman may suspect but cannot be certain that she is pregnant. Scientific data identify what is necessary for sexual intercourse to result in pregnancy and offer an objective basis for the definition of the beginning of a pregnancy.

The reproductive process starts long before heterosexual intercourse, with the formation of specialized cells called *gametes* contained in the reproductive organs of the woman and the man. The formation of a new human being requires the union of a male gamete, a cell called a *spermatozoon*, with a female gamete, a cell called an *ovum*.

All human cells contain tiny structures called *chromosomes*, which carry all the genetic information that is unique to each individual and that contributes to define his or her identity as a person. Gametes are different from all other cells in that they contain only one-half of the chromosomes that are present in the other cells of the body. Human cells have twenty-three different types of chromosomes, named chromosome 1 through 23. Each cell has two of each of the twenty-three types of chromosomes, or a total of forty-six chromosomes, with the exception of the *gametes*, which have only one of each type, or a total of twenty-three chromosomes.

The fusion of the male and female gametes, called *fertilization*, results in the formation of one cell that contains twenty-three pairs of chromosomes (a total of forty-six chromosomes), half from the mother and half from the father. This new cell, called a *zygote*—which results from fertilization and has a complete, new chromosomal identity—has the potential to multiply and become an *embryo*, then a *fetus*, and ultimately a new person.

For fertilization to occur, a number of processes must normally take place. Semen ejaculated by the male, containing millions of spermatozoa, must be deposited in the *vagina* during sexual intercourse. Spermatozoa have great mobility, and the female genital tract possesses mechanisms for the transportation of the gametes to enable spermatozoa to travel from the vagina, through the *cervix of the uterus*, into the *uterine cavity*, and then along the *fallopian tubes* that terminate close to the *ovaries*.

It is in the tubes that a spermatozoon may find and penetrate a female gamete and start the fertilization process.

The period of time from the first day of menstruation until the day before the first day of the next menstruation is called a *menstrual cycle*. In about 90 percent of menstrual cycles in normal women, one of the ovaries delivers one mature ovum into one of the tubes, in the process called *ovulation*. Although ovulation usually occurs at about the middle of the menstrual cycle, it can occur at any time from day 10 through day 24, counting from the first day of menstrual bleeding.

The ovum's capability of being fertilized is a state that lasts for no longer than twenty-four hours. Consequently, fertilization is possible during only one day of each menstrual cycle, the day a woman ovulates. It is important to note, however, that spermatozoa can penetrate and fertilize an ovum up to the sixth day after being deposited in the vagina. Consequently, fertilization can occur only when sexual intercourse has taken place within the five days preceding ovulation (Wilcox, Weinberg, and Baird, 1995).

Furthermore, of the millions of spermatozoa deposited in the vagina, a few hundred reach the fallopian tubes in a few minutes, but animal experimentation shows that these spermatozoa are not capable of fertilizing an ovum (Chang, 1984). Hundreds of thousands remain for some time in the uterine cervix, protected by the *cervical mucus*. These spermatozoa constitute a reservoir from which successive groups continue their journey into the uterus and then into the tubes during the subsequent hours and days. Some spermatozoa from each group adhere for hours to the cells lining the tubes, where they acquire the capacity to fertilize, a process called *capacitation* (Töpfer-Petersen, Petrounkina, and Ekhlasi-Hundrieser, 2000). They maintain this capacity for only a few hours or even minutes after they detach from the wall of the tube to look for the ovum. When a capacitated spermatozoon finds a capable ovum, and if the environment is appropriate, fertilization can proceed (Croxatto, 2002a). The fusion of the gametes takes several hours to complete, and the resulting *zygote* then starts to multiply in the interior of the tube.

Three or four days after fertilization, a cluster of eight to ten cells enters the uterine cavity and, still immersed in the liquid that exists in the genital tract, continues to multiply (Ortiz and Croxatto, 1990). By the seventh day, when the number has increased to about two hundred cells, the process of *implantation* begins: The cluster of cells, now called a *blastocyst*, penetrates the inner layer of the uterine cavity, called the *endometrium*, and settles there. This process of implantation takes about four days to complete. Although each cell in the blastocyst contains identical genetic information, only a few of the central cells will constitute the future embryo. The remaining 90 percent will form the placenta and the membranes that will envelop the fetus.

It is only at the time of implantation that a woman's body clearly recognizes that a new individual is developing within her. At this time some of the implanted cells start to produce a hormone called *HCG*, which enters the woman's blood stream, reaches her ovary, and affects its function. The presence of HCG interferes with the mechanism that triggers menstruation, which results from a decrease in the production of the ovarian hormones, *estrogens* and *progesterone*. Instead, HCG stimulates the ovary to increase the production of hormones, particularly progesterone, which protects the embryo and allows it to develop.

It is worth noting that these complex circumstances explain the relative inefficiency of the reproductive process. In fact, of one hundred normal couples who, at the peak of their fertility, have sexual intercourse several times per month, only twenty-five women will become pregnant the first month, and only another 25 percent of the remaining seventy-five women (or about nineteen women) will become pregnant the following month. Pregnancies will continue to occur at the same rate in subsequent months.

The 25 percent pregnancy rate each month results from the combination of two processes: each month, fertilization will occur in only half the women, and among the women in whom fertilization is successful, 50 percent of the fertilized eggs will fail to implant or will be eliminated soon after implantation. Certainly all these percentages are approximations that will vary according to several factors, such as age and previous disease of one or both partners .

From Embryo to Newborn Baby

After successful implantation, the embryo continues to grow, and the cells continue to become organized for different functions—first by further separating into those that will form the fetus itself and those, such as the placenta and the membranes that surround the fetus, that will feed and protect it. A few days after implantation is completed—about fourteen or fifteen days after fertilization and more or less coinciding with the cessation of menstruation—when there are a few thousand cells that measure under 1.5 millimeters, the *primitive streak* is formed.

Under the microscope the primitive streak is seen as a piling of cells that form a line from which a fetus may eventually develop. Rarely, two primitive streaks are formed, and from them identical *twins* may develop. Twinning can start earlier, but it can occur no later in the reproductive process. Furthermore, at this stage of the reproductive process, it is also possible that none of the cells that resulted from the multiplication of the zygote will develop into an embryo, no primitive streak will occur, and hence no new individual will form. In medicine this phenomenon results in what is called a *blighted ovum*. Consequently, before the appearance of the primitive streak, at about the time of the first missed menstrual period, the product of fertilization is referred to as a *pre-embryo*, and after the appearance of the primitive streak, it is known as an *embryo*.

The embryo continues to grow, and during the fourth week following fertilization (about six weeks after the last menstruation), the developing heart starts to beat and the buds of what will become the extremities appear. Because the length of pregnancy is usually considered by physicians and by laypersons to be the number of weeks or months after the last menstruation, that is the designation we will use.

By the end of ten weeks of pregnancy, the embryo measures about three centimeters, and the early expression of all essential external and internal structures is present. Biologists refer to stages from this point on as phases of *fetal* development. By the end of the first trimester of pregnancy (twelve to thirteen weeks after the last menstruation), the genitalia of the fetus start to differentiate into female or male, and the face acquires a human appearance. This is also the earliest point at which a microscopic connection between neural cells has been described in the zone where, months later, the brain cortex will develop (Sass, 1994). The fetus continues to grow and develop, and about four or five months after her last menstruation, the pregnant woman begins to feel the movements of the fetus in her womb, traditionally known as *quickening*.

Growth and development of a normal fetus continue until birth, and beyond birth in the case of a normal infant. During this process, the fetus reaches another milestone—*viability*, or the time when the fetus is able to survive outside the woman's body. The timeframe for viability has changed with the progress of neonatology, but even with the advances made in neonatal intensive care, it is currently accepted that no child born before twenty-three weeks of gestation will survive. Consequently, WHO defines the perinatal period as commencing at twenty-two completed weeks of gestation, when birth weight is approximately five hundred grams (WHO, 1977). Pregnancies that end before this time are therefore defined as abortions, whereas those that terminate from the twenty-third week on are considered premature births. The International Federation of Gynecology and Obstetrics (FIGO) Committee for the Ethical Aspects of Human Reproduction and Women's Health has endorsed this distinction, adding that the stages of development between twenty-two and twenty-eight weeks of gestation should be considered the "threshold of viability" (Schenker, 1997).

The survival of babies born after twenty-two weeks but before twenty-eight weeks of gestation—during which time the average newborn weighs less than one kilogram—is contingent upon very sophisticated and specialized medical facilities, and those who survive often suffer severe and permanent disabilities (Kitchen et al., 1985; Duggan, 2002). In the absence of a specialized care center, most babies born during this period, particularly before twenty-six weeks of gestation, will die (Schenker, 1997). The chances of survival continue to increase as pregnancy progresses; however, even with full-term deliveries, survival depends on care received, and fetuses with severe malformations, such as anencephaly (the lack of the upper portions of the brain), do not survive more than a few hours after birth.

The Beginning of Pregnancy and of a New Individual

The question frequently raised in public discussions is "When does human life begin?" This is the wrong question: Human life is a continuum through generations, and all the components involved in the reproductive process—at all stages, from the gametes onward—are human and are alive. A more pertinent question is "When does pregnancy start, and when does a new individual begin within the reproductive process?" Commonly, however, the wrong question is followed by the wrong answer: that life begins at conception.

We have carefully avoided confusing the issue by using the word *conception* in our description of the reproductive process. According to the *Oxford Dictionary, to conceive* means "to become pregnant." Consequently, the American College of Obstetrics and Gynecology has defined *conception* as synonymous with *implantation*; for many, however, it means "fertilization," and in the past it has even been used to refer to the act of sexual intercourse that resulted in the pregnancy. Frequently, the term *conception* is used loosely, without a precise biological meaning, and in some religious discussions it is even used to imply the time of ensoulment, when the soul is believed to enter the new individual.

Consequently, in order to avoid confusion, we will not use the word *conception*, to define the beginning of pregnancy or of a new individual.

Definitions are arbitrary agreements based on logical thought. WHO and FIGO have defined *pregnancy* as beginning with implantation (Schenker and Cain, 1999). This definition is based on the logic that pregnancy is something that happens to the woman and before implantation her body seems unaware of the presence of the pre-embryo. In addition, earlier stages of the reproductive process frequently do not result in pregnancy. Moreover, the in vitro process of fertilization in a laboratory dish followed by the very early stages of pre-embryo development, a frequent occurrence in assisted reproductive services, is never considered pregnancy. In short, in accordance with WHO and FIGO, *we define pregnancy as the stage of the reproductive process during which the body of the woman and the developing new individual interlace with each other, which starts at implantation and ends when an abortion or a birth takes place.*

A different rationale would apply if the question were: When do cells with a new chromosome identity start to exist? In that case the answer would be that they begin to exist at fertilization. Although it could also be said that the zygote, the cell that results from fertilization, has the potential to become a new individual and—if it implants and develops normally—eventually a new person, the logic of considering the zygote a new individual is questionable. As Professor Croxatto commented, "A seed may become a tree and eggs may become chickens, but a seed is not a tree and an egg is not a chicken" (personal communication, 2001). Another reason for rejecting the idea that an individual begins at fertilization is that a zygote can be the origin of more than a single individual, when, for unknown reasons, its development results in a multiple pregnancy. This twinning capacity, as we have seen, is possible up to two weeks after fertilization.

Based on these biological explanations, many biologists—and even a prominent Catholic theologian (Ford, 1988)—maintain that the beginning of a new individual cannot be designated before the primitive streak appears (about fourteen days after fertilization and after implantation is complete). For this reason, as we have seen, early stages of the reproductive process are referred to as pre-embryonic development.

Another milestone occurs in the development of the fetus when the maturation of the central nervous system has reached the point where all bodily functions are integrated and it is possible to feel pain and eventually develop all cognitive functions. After reviewing similar proposals made by physicians, theologians, and other philosophers, prominent Catholic philosopher Hans-Martin Sass recommended that—in parallel with the generally accepted legal and ethical definition of *death* as "brain death"—legal protection of the life of the fetus begin when there is biological evidence of "brain life" (Sass, 1994). In his own words, "The moral assessment of maturation and cessation of neuro-neuronal functioning, based on biblical, philosophical, and theological tradition, favors a Uniform Determination of Life Protection Act, legally protecting personal life (animate life) from the beginning of brain functioning (brain life) to its end (brain death)" (Sass, 1994, p. 58).

Sass considers the beginning of brain life to occur at the end of twelve weeks of gestation, or seventy days after fertilization, when the first connections (synapses) among neural cells appear at the site where the cerebral cortex will develop. He recognizes the neuroscientific consensus that there is no constant, well-organized brain activity until at least twenty-two to twenty-eight weeks and that permanent electroencephalographic activity is detectable only after thirty-two weeks, but he prefers a more conservative interpretation to facilitate a broader consensus.

Sass's interpretation parallels imminent death and imminent life. It is generally accepted that, in spite of the persistence of other biological activities, the cessation of brain activity defines imminent death. Similarly, according to Sass, before brain activity is possible, in spite of the existence of a heartbeat and other biological functions, the fetus has only imminent life.

Ectopic Pregnancy

During the normal reproductive process, the developing pre-embryo implants in the inner surface of the uterus, called the *endometrium*. In some abnormal conditions, usually as a result of partial obstruction of the fallopian tubes, the fertilized egg does not reach the uterine cavity and implants in the tube or, more rarely, in the surface of the ovary or in the *peritoneum*, the membrane that covers the abdominal cavity. These cases are, respectively, a *tubal*, an *ovarian*, and an *abdominal ectopic pregnancy*. Ovarian and abdominal pregnancies are so rare that in normal medical jargon they are referred to by their specific names and the term *ectopic pregnancy* is used to describe a tubal pregnancy.

In a small percentage of tubal pregnancies, the pre-embryo fails to grow and can be reabsorbed spontaneously (Yao and Tulandi, 1997). In most cases, the growth of the embryo dilates the tube until it ruptures, and the rupture of the tube causes an internal hemorrhage. It is not uncommon for this to result in maternal death, particularly in localities where access to emergency surgery is unavailable. Ectopic pregnancy can be diagnosed before rupture and treated with conservative surgery consisting of opening the tube, removing the embryonic tissue, and re-suturing the tube to preserve the woman's fertility. Emergency treatment after rupture invariably means surgical removal of the tube.

Defining Induced Abortion

The definition of *abortion* as simply the termination of pregnancy is inadequate, because this includes any birth before the completion of normal gestation. The difference between abortion and premature birth is viability. The FIGO Ethics Committee defines induced abortion as "the termination of pregnancy using drugs or surgical intervention after implantation and before the conceptus [the product of conception] has become independently viable" (Schenker and Cain, 1999, p.318). As we have noted, WHO has established viability at twenty-two completed weeks of gestation, or a weight of five hundred grams. Consequently, the termination of pregnancy when the fetus is below that limit is defined as an abortion, and the termination of a pregnancy when the fetus is above that limit is considered premature birth.

Safe and Unsafe Abortion

Safe abortion and *unsafe abortion* are common terms that are used frequently in international documents. WHO (1992) defines *unsafe abortion* as "a procedure for terminating an unwanted pregnancy either by persons lacking the necessary skills or in an environment lacking the minimal medical standards, or both" (AbouZhar and Ahman, 1998, p.276). In contrast, a medical or surgical abortion performed by a well-trained professional with the necessary resources and in a suitable medical environment is considered to be a safe abortion because there is little risk to the woman. The maternal mortality observed with safe abortion is no more than one in one hundred thousand procedures, and there are few complications. In fact, if the abortion is performed early in the pregnancy (up to twelve weeks), the associated morbidity and mortality are lower than those of a normal full-term delivery.

Most unsafe abortions are performed in countries where they are legally restricted. However, some occur in countries where abortion is legal but the conditions under which the procedure is performed are inadequate. It is also noteworthy that many safe abortions are performed in countries where abortion is legally restricted. Therefore, it is important that the usage of the terms *safe abortion* and *unsafe abortion* be kept distinct from the usage of the terms *legal abortion* and *illegal abortion*.

Methods of Pregnancy Termination

Since ancient times, a wide range of methods has been used to induce abortions, from very primitive procedures to modern surgical techniques and medications.

Traditionally and even today, a popular method of unsafe abortion has been the introduction of a solid, pointed object through the uterine cervix to cause the membrane protecting the embryo/fetus to rupture and allow a pathway for infection. The woman's own body then rejects the infected embryo or fetus. A number of different potions and herbal teas have also been used with questionable effectiveness. A popular traditional method used mostly in Asia is to massage the pregnant woman's abdomen forcefully. All of these methods commonly result in incomplete abortions with severe uterine or generalized infections, requiring emergency care to save the woman's life.

The vast majority of maternal deaths caused by induced abortion result from the performance of these primitive procedures under unhygienic conditions. Fortunately, an increasing number of abortions are performed using more modern techniques classified into two main categories: (1) instrumental evacuation of the uterine cavity through the cervix, either by dilatation and curettage (D & C) or, preferably, by intrauterine vacuum aspiration and (2) the administration of medications, also referred to as pharmacological abortions. Other methods, such as the injection of substances into the uterus or the surgical removal of the fetus through the abdomen (micro-cesareans), have been abandoned because of the higher risk of complications and death (Cates et al. 1977).

Until the second half of the twentieth century, D & C was the most common—indeed virtually the only—method used. D & C, or the introduction of metallic objects of increasing diameters to force cervical dilation that then allows the introduction of a sharp curette, is now generally used from six to fourteen weeks of pregnancy. The curette, a long instrument that ends in a small hollowed spoon with sharp borders, is introduced into the uterus, and the walls of the uterine cavity are scraped with the sharp border of the "spoon" to systematically remove the tissues adhering to the interior surface of the uterus. Curettes come in many sizes, measured by the diameter of the spoon and ranging from 2 mm to about 1 cm. The size of the curette needed depends on the number of weeks of pregnancy and the cervical dilatation that can be achieved.

Beyond fourteen weeks, a similar procedure—dilatation and evacuation, or D & E—can be performed. D & E requires greater cervical dilatation, to allow the use of both a curette with a greater diameter and forceps for the removal of fetal parts. This procedure requires greater skill than D & C and involves higher risk. Fortunately, most abortions are performed during the first trimester.

Vacuum aspiration, a method of emptying the uterus introduced by the Chinese, does not require cervical dilatation when performed up to six weeks of pregnancy, because a plastic tube that is small in diameter is introduced through the cervix to extract the uterine content, which is minimal and soft. For abortions between seven and twelve weeks, vacuum aspiration requires cervical dilatation, but the uterine evacuation is faster, causes less bleeding, and is associated with fewer complications and less pain than with the D & C (Tietze and Lewit, 1972; Edelman, Brenner, and Berger, 1974; Cates et al., 1977; Hart and Macharper, 1986). The vacuum action can be produced by an electrical pump, but in recent decades most of these procedures have been performed using manual vacuum aspiration (MVA) with a disposable syringe and plastic tubing. Simplification of the procedure and the use of state-of-the-art equipment have lowered the risk of complications and have enabled well-trained non-medical providers to perform the procedure safely and effectively. Currently, there is general agreement that vacuum aspiration should replace D & C (Greenslade et al., 1993).

Pharmacological abortions first became possible in the 1980s, when French researchers (Baulieu and Rosenblum, 1990) succeeded in developing RU486, a molecule very similar to progesterone (which is necessary for an early pregnancy to proceed) that blocks the action of the ovarian hormone. RU486, when given alone within the first seven weeks of pregnancy, causes an abortion in 80 percent of cases (Baulieu, 1985). This antiprogesterone drug, which has been given the name mifepristone, is currently used in combination with a prostaglandin, which softens and dilates the cervix and stimulates uterine contractions. When a prostaglandin is administered forty-eight hours after mifepristone, effectiveness is raised to 96 percent (Peyron et al., 1993; Ulmann and Silvestre, 1994; Hollander, 1995).

Since the 1960s, prostaglandins have also been used alone, administered intravaginally or intracervically, to induce abortion (Karim and Filshie, 1970a; Karim and Filshie, 1970b; Karim, 1971); however, unpleasant side effects, high cost, and instability at normal temperature (requiring refrigeration) have limited their use. In the late 1980s, a new synthetic prostaglandin for the treatment or prevention of gastric peptic ulcers was registered. The new synthetic prostaglandin, misoprostol, is stable at room temperature and therefore easier to store and dispense. Many clinical studies have shown misoprostol to be at least as effective as other prostaglandins for abortion induction, and it has become part of the most commonly used mifepristone-plus-prostaglandin regimen (Wong et al., 1998; Schaff et al., 2000; WHO, 2000; Schaff, Fielding, and Westhoff, 2001).

In addition, misoprostol alone, administered in dosages of 800 mcg by the vaginal route, has proven to be close to 90 percent effective in inducing abortions (Carbonell et al., 1999; Bugalho et al., 2000). Its advantage over mifepristone is that it is effective at any gestational age and requires lower doses as pregnancy advances; at full term, only a 25-mcg dose is required to induce labor (ACOG, 2000). Misoprostol when used alone has a lower effectiveness than when it is used in combination with mifepristone, but it is also associated with fewer side effects, such as nausea and vomiting (Jain, Meckstroth, and Mishell, 1999; Kain et al., 2002).

The mifepristone-plus-misoprostol regimen is effective up to nine weeks of pregnancy. Vacuum aspiration can be used to terminate pregnancies up to twelve weeks. D & C can be used up to fourteen weeks of pregnancy. For second-trimester abortion, misoprostol is the preferred method.

In general, the more advanced the pregnancy is at the time of abortion, the greater the risk of complications and death (Atrash et al., 1987; Lawson et al., 1994). Most abortions are performed within the first twelve weeks of pregnancy, but the number performed later—particularly in cases of severe fetal malformation or risk to the life of the woman—is not insignificant. In such cases, misoprostol offers the great advantage of being highly effective after twelve weeks, inducing abortion with characteristics that mimic miscarriage.

"Partial-Birth" Abortion

The abortion debate has frequently been complicated by the manipulation of words and images. A good example is the term *"partial-birth" abortion,* which was created in 1995 to introduce a law intended to restrict abortion rights in the United States by making a specific surgical procedure illegal. The gruesome image of the head of a fetus being partially destroyed to facilitate its extraction was theatrically presented in Congress.

"Partial-birth" abortion is required only under extremely rare circumstances: very late in pregnancy, in locations without surgical facilities, in order to save the life of the woman. The procedure is usually used in cases of obstructed labor, where a deformation of the pelvis prevents the fetus's head from advancing, a circumstance that can cause rupture of the uterus and death for both the woman and the fetus. Although it may be necessary to perform the procedure on a normal, viable fetus in remote clinics in developing countries, there is virtually no justification for its use under these circumstances in developed regions of the world. It is worthwhile noting that these cases do not fall into the category of abortion, since they occur during the third trimester of pregnancy and up to full-term delivery. Declaring this procedure illegal was a surreptitious method of restricting abortions in general. Although it was never precisely defined, the term *partial-birth abortion* became an ideological banner. The implication was that the law intended to prohibit only this lamentable procedure, but the vague language would have opened the door to legal action against many, perhaps all, types of abortion. The so-called Partial-Birth Abortion Ban Act "was twice vetoed by President Clinton [and] the US Supreme Court ruled a similar Nebraska law unconstitutional because it criminalized abortion procedures prior to fetal viability and regardless of the implications for the woman's health" (Cohen, 2002, p. 1). Such conscious efforts to mislead the public with false information distort the real question. Unfortunately, in 2003 the legal proposal was revived by a new political majority in the U.S. Congress and an administration that seemed committed to what was called in the title of a January 12, 2003, *New York Times* editorial "The War against Women." Congress passed a new version of the law, which was then signed by President George W. Bush in November 2003. As an editorial in the *New England Journal of Medicine* aptly observed, the language is still subject to interpretation, and it will be up to the courts to determine its constitutionality. (Greene and Ecker, 2004).

Menstrual Regulation

Menstrual regulation is a medical procedure related to abortion that may or may not involve a very early pregnancy termination. It consists of the evacuation of the uterine content of a woman who has a short delay in menstruation (usually no more than two weeks), without determining whether or not she is pregnant. This practice originated with the introduction of vacuum aspiration at a time when early pregnancy tests were not available. In most cases, the woman is pregnant, but she may prefer not to know and to maintain her belief that the procedure was performed only as a menstrual delay for moral, religious, or cultural reasons (Nations et al., 1997). In addition, both the physician and the woman may prefer this procedure for its legal convenience in countries with restrictive legislation. Because the procedure requires little if any cervical dilatation, it can be performed in the physician's office without anesthesia, thus facilitating privacy and maintaining the appearance that it was not an abortion.

The term *menstrual regulation* has now been expanded to include the termination of pregnancies up to twelve weeks, as long as the procedure can be carried out by vacuum aspiration and with local anesthesia. At these later stages, both the physician and the woman know that a pregnancy exists, but—particularly in some Muslim countries, where abortion is legally restricted but early termination of pregnancy is not disallowed in the teachings of the predominant religion—the use of the term *menstrual regulation* serves as a political strategy (Kabir, 1989).

The many terms defined here are used frequently in the following chapters, and the definition or explanation provided above will not be repeated.

3
The Magnitude
of Induced Abortion

It is practically impossible to know how many induced abortions occur in the world every year because reliable data are available for only a relatively small number of countries. One of the most complete analyses of the global incidence of abortion, a study by Stanley. K. Henshaw, Susheela Singh, and Taylor Haas (1999), identified only twenty-eight countries with data "believed to be complete."

It is easy to understand the lack of data on abortions in countries where it is legally restricted, since reporting abortion may result in severe consequences for both woman and provider. Consequently, these countries keep no official statistics, and their estimates on the incidence of abortion are primarily based on the number of women who are treated in the health care system for abortion complications. In many countries, however, these statistics include only women who are treated in the public health system, and even these cases are often underreported.

Studies that involve interviewing representative samples of the population are also used, although it is well known that these figures significantly under-represent the true numbers (Barreto et al., 1992; Osis et al., 1996; Jagannathan, 2001). Several innovative methods have been developed to elicit more complete reporting of abortion, but there are good reasons to believe that even the best methods fail to obtain an accurate representation (Barreto et al., 1992).

The best data are obtained from countries where abortion is legal under broad circumstances and where accurate and complete statistical data are collected and recorded. Official statistics even for countries such as the United States, however, are frequently incomplete (Henshaw et al., 1998). Some of the most populated countries, in which a large proportion of the world's abortions are performed, such as the Russian Federation, India, and China, also have problems in under-reporting. The best data from Russia are provided by the Ministry of Health, but they do not include abortions performed in the facilities of other ministries. According to Henshaw, Singh, and Haas (1999), the data from China do not include pharmacologically induced abortions using mifepristone, which may reach a million per year. The fact that only a small fraction of abortions are performed within the current legal framework of India's Medical Termination of Pregnancy (MTP) Act leads us to the conclusion that the data from India also grossly underreport the incidence of abortion (Khan, Barge, and Philip, 1996).

Worldwide Estimations

The analysis by Henshaw, Singh, and Haas (1999) estimated that a total of 46 million abortions were performed in 1995 but acknowledged that, given the unreliability of the data, the number could be as low as 42 million or as high as 50 million. WHO accepts 46 million as the best estimate (WHO, 1997, 2004). According to Henshaw, Singh, and Haas (1999), 26 percent of all pregnancies, not including miscarriages and stillbirths, terminate in abortion each year. This means that one out of every four pregnancies worldwide is voluntarily terminated annually, a statistic that illustrates the enormous dimension of the problem.

Another way of expressing the magnitude of abortion occurrence is to relate the number of abortions to the number of women who could have an abortion, in what is called a rate. The abortion rate is calculated using the number of women of childbearing age, instead of the number of pregnancies, as the basis on which the magnitude of the problem is estimated. The rate shows what percentage of all women of childbearing age will have an induced abortion in a single year. Because the probability of pregnancy is much lower before age fifteen and after age forty-four, demographers commonly (though not always) use ages fifteen to forty-four as the interval that defines *childbearing age*.

Worldwide, the rate of induced abortion is about thirty-five per thousand women between ages fifteen and forty-four. This means that, globally, one out of every twenty-eight women within that age range has an abortion each year.

Regional Differences in Induced Abortion

The largest number of abortions, about 27 million, occurs in Asia, followed by Europe, with 8 million; Africa, with 5 million; Latin America, with 4 million; North America, with 1.5 million; and Oceania, with 0.1 million (Singh and Wulf, 1994; Singh et al., 1997; Huntington et al., 1998; Henshaw, Singh, and Haas, 1999). These numbers are obviously influenced by the uneven distribution of the population. Asia has the largest number of abortions because it is also the most populated region of the world. A better view of the risk of induced abortion is seen by comparing the rates.

The abortion rate is highest in Europe, with forty-eight per thousand women (48/1,000), followed by Latin America (37/1,000), Asia and Africa (33/1,000), North America (22/1,000), and Oceania (21/1,000). Regional rates, however, conceal vast differences within each continent. The greatest contrast is between eastern and western Europe with, respectively, the highest and the lowest rates in the world.

The abortion rate in eastern Europe may be as high as ninety per thousand women of childbearing age. This high number is influenced by a culture of small families, compounded by both the poor quality of contraceptive methods and inadequate access to them, on one hand, and traditionally free and easily accessible abortions, on the other hand (David, 1982). Although abortion appears to have become more difficult to access in recent years, it is apparently still more accessible than effective contraceptive methods (Stephen, 2002).

The situation is reversed in western Europe, which has the lowest rate in the world, with eleven induced abortions per thousand women between the ages of fifteen and forty-four (Henshaw, Singh, and Haas, 1999). Four countries in this region present reliable data, each with an abortion rate below ten per thousand: Belgium, Germany, the Netherlands, and Switzerland.

In both eastern and western Europe, the large majority of induced abortions are legal. The exceptions are some countries from the former Soviet Union, where some women prefer the privacy of clandestine abortion to the embarrassment and inconvenience associated with the use of public health services.

In contrast, the great majority of induced abortions in Latin America are illegal —with the exception of Cuba, Guyana, and some English-speaking Caribbean nations. Nevertheless, the abortion rate in some Latin American countries (such as Chile, where abortion is not permitted under any circumstances) is estimated to be as high as fifty per thousand. The highest rate in Latin America, however, was observed in Cuba, with almost seventy-eight abortions per thousand women of childbearing age (Henshaw, Singh, and Haas, 1999). Cuba suffers conditions very similar to those in the former Soviet states, conditions that are aggravated by the commercial blockade implemented by the United States. Consequently, access to contraceptive methods of good quality is limited, whereas access to menstrual regulation or later abortion is not (Hardy et al., 1990; Alvarez, 1992). Recent statistics from the Cuban Ministry of Health indicate, however, that the number of abortions and the abortion rate peaked in 1986, at 162,000 abortions, or 50.6 per 1,000 women of childbearing age, and decreased by more than half in 2001, to 70,000 abortions, or a rate of 21.2 per 1,000 women (Ministerio de Salud Pública de Cuba, 2001). These numbers have to be corrected because they do not include menstrual regulations; however, even if there were as many menstrual regulations as abortions, it is unlikely that the present rate for Cuba is any greater than for other Latin American countries where abortion is either illegal or severely restricted.

The highest abortion rate in the Asian continent is registered in the southeastern region (40/1,000). This region includes Vietnam, which appears to have the highest abortion rate in the world, probably as high as 110 per 1,000, including legal and illegal abortions in a proportion of 3:1 (Henshaw, Singh, and Haas, 1999). The estimated rate for eastern Asia, which comprises China, Japan, Mongolia, Hong Kong, North Korea, and South Korea, is close to that of Latin America (36/1,000). Personal communication between the authors and Chinese health and population officials indicates that the abortion rate in China is rapidly declining, from thirty per thousand women of childbearing age in the first half of the 1990s to approximately 20 per 1,000 in recent years. This drop in the abortion rate can be attributed in part to the recent progressive substitution of the highly effective Copper T-380 IUD in place of relatively inert models traditionally used in a country where the IUD is the most common method of contraception (Kaufman, 1993). The estimated abortion rate for South Central Asia, which includes such sizable countries as India, Pakistan, and Bangladesh, is the lowest in the continent (28/1,000), though this rate may be underestimated (see later discussion).

Estimations for the continent of Africa prove most difficult. Contrary to Asia, where most of the population lives in countries in which abortion is legal, Africa comprises nations that, for the most part, legally restrict induced abortion. Dividing the continent into regions, the highest rate (40/1,000) is found in the eastern region, which includes Burundi, Ethiopia, Kenya, Madagascar, Malawi, Mauritius, Mozambique, Rwanda, Somalia, Uganda, Tanzania, Zambia, and Zimbabwe (Henshaw, Singh, and Haas, 1999; Ethiopian Society of Obstetrics and Gynecology, 2000).

The lowest rate (17/1,000) is observed in northern Africa, comprising Algeria, Egypt, Libya, Morocco, Sudan, and Tunisia. Tunisia, one of the few countries in Africa where abortion is legal, is the country with the lowest abortion rate, only eleven per thousand women of childbearing age. This is another good example of the lack of correlation between legality and abortion rate. southern Africa (comprising Botswana, Lesotho, Namibia, Swaziland, and the Republic of South Africa), the least populated region on the continent, also has a relatively low rate (19/1,000), with abortion being legal in the largest of these countries, the Republic of South Africa.

The estimated abortion rate for the United States was 22.9 per 1,000 in 1996 (Henshaw, 1998), well above the western European rate. This is not very surprising, considering that access to contraception is more difficult for large segments of the U.S. population than it is for western Europeans. In addition, sex education begins very early in western Europe and is virtually universal, whereas in the United States it is limited and ideologically restricted.

The number of and rates of induced abortion do not tell the whole story, however, because pregnancy termination can be carried out in a wide range of conditions in various parts of the world or among different groups within the same country. Therefore, it is important to analyze regional variations in the incidence of unsafe abortion.

Regional Differences in Unsafe Abortion

Safety is closely correlated to the legality of abortion: Most illegal abortions are performed under unsafe conditions, and most legal abortions are performed under safe conditions (although there are a number of exceptions to this rule, as explained in Chapter 4. The terms *safe abortion* and *unsafe abortion* are used to distinguish the difference in risk to women who have induced abortions.

According to Henshaw, Singh, and Haas (1999), of the 46 million induced abortions estimated for 1995, 26 million corresponded to generally safe legal abortions and 20 million to mostly unsafe illegal abortions. In our judgment, these estimates of the number of unsafe abortions are conservative for some parts of the world. Although their analysis was very careful and detailed, we have reasons to believe that the authors did not fully correct for the missing data. One example is the estimate of 8.4 million induced abortions, including 6.5 million unsafe abortions in South Central Asia. This number contrasts with the Shah Committee estimate of 6 million unsafe abortions performed outside the official health system in India alone, for 1991 (Chhabra, 1996). It is difficult to believe that there were a mere five hundred thousand unsafe abortions in the other twelve countries in the South Central Asia region combined, including Afghanistan, Bangladesh, Bhutan, Iran, Kazakhstan, Kyrgyzstan, Nepal, Pakistan, Sri Lanka, Tajikistan, Turkmenistan, and Uzbekistan. Moreover, the Shah Committee data refer to 1991. More recent estimates indicate a sharp increase in induced abortions in India—the majority of which were performed in unsafe conditions—mounting to 10 million in 2001. This figure is almost twice the estimate of Henshaw, Singh, and Haas for all thirteen countries of the South Central Asia region (Jain, 2001). Thus, it is quite possible that at the present time the number of unsafe abortions is equal to the number of safe abortions in the world.

Safe and unsafe abortions, however, are not homogeneously distributed throughout the different regions of the world. Developed countries make up more than 20 percent of the world's population but only 5 percent of unsafe abortions. This incongruity occurs because abortions in developed countries are mostly legal and safe, whereas abortions in developing countries, with the exception of China, are mostly illegal and unsafe. India is another densely populated country where abortion is legal, but in India the vast majority of induced abortions are still performed in unsafe conditions outside the official health system (Chhabra, 1996).

More recent estimates of unsafe abortion rates by region show that the highest incidence per thousand women between ages fifteen and forty-nine is in Latin America (26/1,000), followed by Africa (22/1,000), and Asia (11/1,000), the rate for Asia being influenced by the inclusion of China. Considering regions within each continent, the highest rate is found in South America (30/1,000), followed by eastern Africa (29/1,000), western Africa (24/1,000), and South Central Asia (20/1,000). The rate of unsafe abortion in the more developed regions is only two per thousand (Ahman and Shah, 2002).

As we will see in the following chapter, these differences in abortion safety account for a huge imbalance between the effect on the lives of women in developing countries and the effect on the lives of women in the more developed world.

4
Consequences of Unsafe Abortion

Roberta was a very pretty girl, the younger of two daughters of a hard-working man who owned a modest car repair shop in a working-class neighborhood of a large city. Although her mother, a housewife, was almost completely illiterate, both of Roberta's parents wanted a better life for their two daughters and were committed to providing them with the best possible education.

When Roberta was fifteen years old, her eighteen-year-old sister became pregnant by her boyfriend, who was the same age. Her father was furious and rapidly arranged for the wedding before the pregnancy became physically evident. The parents of the boy were equally committed to keeping up appearances and were completely in favor of the marriage. Because Roberta and her sister shared a room, and the boy was an only child and had more space at his home than Roberta's sister, the new couple decided to live with the boy's family. Roberta's sister left school and gave birth to the baby, but less than a year later—unable to tolerate her mother-in-law's continuous recriminations and her husband's indifference and verbal abuse—she returned to her parents' home. Although her mother and father occasionally reminded her of her indiscretion, they also treated the baby and her with love and compassion. Still, her old life of school, friends, and occasional parties was gone forever.

This was a lesson for Roberta, who promised herself that she would never make the same mistake as her sister. She had no idea, however, that she was about to fall in love. Ricardo was sweet and tender. He made her feel important, beautiful, and loved, and Roberta would do anything for him. Although she had promised herself that she would abstain from sex, one summer afternoon Roberta and Ricardo went hiking on a nearby mountain and stopped to rest in a beautiful, rather secluded spot. Their mutual caresses became increasingly intimate, and they ended up making love, both for the first time. Although Roberta did not have an orgasm, she loved the pleasure she was able to give Ricardo and the feeling of the most intimate union of their bodies and souls. In the weekends that followed, she could not stop herself from repeating the act over and over again. Roberta tried to avoid making love during her fertile period, but she wasn't sure when it was and it was hard to curb their passion.

Inevitably, Roberta became pregnant, but she knew that she could not repeat her sister's experience. She knew that neither her parents nor her boyfriend's parents would be able to tolerate the situation, and she did not want to give her parents, who had already suffered enough, another cause for worry. She decided not even to tell her boyfriend; instead she asked around until she found a woman who would perform an inexpensive abortion. The procedure was extremely painful. Roberta left the abortionist's house bleeding heavily, and when she got home, she closed herself in her room, saying that she had a bad stomachache, and tried to avoid her mother's sharp eye. But Roberta continued to bleed and had such severe abdominal pain that her sister finally noticed and went to their mother for help. When they got Roberta to the hospital, she was already very anemic. She had a perforated uterus that required emergency surgery. Despite the infection, the surgeon preserved Roberta's uterus in consideration of her age, in the hope that she would recover. She remained in the intensive care unit for a few days, receiving several blood transfusions and continuous intravenous antibiotics. In a week, she was transferred to the abortion ward. There some very nice women volunteers talked to her about the dangers of abortion and the different methods of contraception. Roberta liked their company and their cheerful manner, but she paid little attention to what they were saying. She was nearly seventeen years old and had already decided that she would never, ever have sex again. Ricardo had disappeared with no explanation and Roberta vowed never to fall in love again. Her parents had been most understanding, and she did not want to disappoint them.

As the reader may already have imagined, less than a year later, in spite of her best intentions, Roberta fell in love again, and the story repeated itself almost exactly. This time, however, Roberta's infection was far more severe. Again, because she was so young and was childless, the surgeons tried to preserve her uterus and at least one fallopian tube and ovary. Unfortunately, after three operations, the doctors could save neither her uterus nor her ovaries. Roberta lost over 40 pounds and was in and out of intensive care for almost two months. Although she seemed near death on several occasions, she managed to survive. Her sad smile combined with an incredible optimism won the admiration of the hospital staff. By the time she finally left the hospital, Roberta had decided that she was going to become a doctor or a nurse. She knew that she would never be able to have children and might never be able to find a husband, so she decided to dedicate her life to caring for others. Everyone hoped that she would succeed in overcoming the tragedy that had touched her life.

Roberta's story illustrates the severe human, social, and economic costs of unsafe abortion: The human cost derives from the physical complications, which can result in the woman's death or several, serious, long term *sequelae* of unsafe abortion. The social cost can result from long-term physical limitations, such as infertility, or from the legal and moral condemnation suffered by women who abort. The economic cost for developing countries, where unsafe abortion prevails, results from the depletion of limited health care resources allocated to women who experience abortion complications, therefore diverting resources from other crucial health requirements of the population.

Maternal Mortality

By far, the most dramatic consequence of induced abortion is that many women pay with their lives. This is the price of the unsafe conditions under which abortions are performed. The hardship experienced by these women and their families is hidden beneath the harsh statistics of the maternal mortality rate.

Maternal mortality is defined as the death of a woman during the period of pregnancy and up to one year after delivery from causes related to the state of pregnancy or aggravated by gestation. It is estimated that about 585,000 maternal deaths occur worldwide every year and that about 13 percent of these deaths are the result of unsafe abortions (WHO, 1997). A more recent UN evaluation estimates that 529,000 women die of maternal causes each year, but the report notes that the margin of error does not permit the conclusion that maternal mortality has decreased in recent years (AbouZhar and Wardlaw, 2003). This means that close to 70,000 women die every year following induced abortion (WHO, 2004). Abortion-related deaths occur predominantly in developing countries, because most illegal and therefore unsafe abortions are performed in these countries and they are performed under more dangerous conditions than in developed countries.

Whereas the risk of death from a safe abortion is about one in a hundred thousand in the United States, the risk of death from an unsafe abortion in a developing country varies between one per hundred and one per thousand. In other words, for a woman in Nigeria or Bolivia, the risk involved in the decision to terminate an unwanted pregnancy is a hundred to a thousand times greater than for a woman making the same decision in the United States (WHO, 1997, 2004). Even within developing countries, the risk of death following induced abortion varies greatly. The incidence of unsafe abortion in Latin America in the late 1980s was forty-one per thousand for women fifteen to forty-nine years old, almost twice the incidence of twenty-six per thousand found in Africa. However, the abortion-related mortality was under fifty per hundred thousand live births in Latin America and over eighty per hundred thousand live births in Africa (WHO, 1993). In other words, women in Africa had fewer abortions but more abortion-related deaths than women in Latin America.

Physical Complications

Abortion-related deaths are just the tip of a broad-based iceberg. Unsafe abortions frequently lead to immediate complications and then long-term consequences. The immediate complications are hemorrhage, infection, traumatic or chemical lesion of the genitals and other organs, and toxic reactions to products ingested or placed in the genitals.

Hemorrhage can lead to acute anemia, shock, and death. Women who have heavy bleeding frequently require an emergency blood transfusion, which in countries with a high prevalence of AIDS and inadequate facilities for testing blood donations, results in a high risk of HIV contamination.

Infections may be limited to the inner surface of the uterus but often travel to the fallopian tubes, the ovaries, and the abdominal cavity, causing pelvic inflammatory disease and even peritonitis. Infections can also disseminate through the blood, leading to sepsis and septic shock. These severe complications can result in death. In fact, among women who request hospital care for abortion complications in some African countries, as many as 7 percent (or one out of every fourteen women) may die (Adewole, 1992).

Women who survive the immediate complications of unsafe abortions often suffer more extended or even long-term consequences through two different paths. First, the treatment required to prevent death frequently includes the removal of the fallopian tubes, the ovaries, and/or the uterus, as it did in *Roberta's* case. A study in South Africa found that 5.4 percent of abortion patients required the removal of the uterus (a hysterectomy) and more than half of these women were childless (Richards et al., 1985). Second, even when these organs do not require removal, inflammation of the tubes frequently leads to their obstruction. Obstructed tubes can result in infertility or, if the obstruction is partial, can lead to an ectopic tubal pregnancy, in which the zygote is implanted in the tube. If the condition is not diagnosed and treated in time, the growth of the embryo will rupture the tube causing severe hemorrhage, which is another frequent cause of death if immediate access to surgical treatment is not available.

In cases of chronic inflammation of the upper genital organs or surgical scars, in addition to the risks of infertility and tubal pregnancy, chronic pelvic pain is common. Continuous lower abdominal pain, exacerbated by certain movements, heavy lifting, and sexual intercourse (when the penis touches the cervix or penetrates too deeply into the vagina) is a frequent occurrence. As we will see, the resulting limitations to movement and activity, and interference with sexual intercourse, may also have severe social consequences (Ladipo, 1989; Liskin, 1992).

Psychological Consequences

During the past twenty years, groups that oppose women's right to abortion have insisted on the existence of a disorder they call abortion trauma syndrome (Speckhard and Rue, 1992), but careful analysis of data has led to the conclusion that the syndrome is more myth than reality (JAMA, 1992).

In recent decades, several reviews of the literature on the psychological consequences of induced abortion have been published (David et al., 1978; Rogers, Stoms, and Phifer, 1989). Although there are some variations in their findings, the common ground is that adverse psychological sequelae occur in only a small percentage of women. In fact, the frequency and severity of adverse psychological effects are much greater among women who are denied abortion and among the children who are born as a result (David et al., 1978; Handy, 1982; Romans-Clarkson, 1989; Dagg, 1991).

Moreover, according to the majority of studies, women who experienced psychological symptoms such as depression following induced abortion had suffered the same symptoms prior to the abortion; or the decision to abort was not their own but rather the result of external pressure, particularly from their partners (Romans-Clarkson, 1989). Psychological symptoms also occur when a wanted pregnancy is terminated after diagnosis of a genetic fetal defect (Adler et al., 1990). In addition, external pressure from a cultural-religious environment that confers strong negative connotation to abortion is also associated with a greater risk of emotional complications from induced abortion (Zolese)

A well designed study compared the incidence of post–induced-abortion psychosis and postpartum psychosis in the same population and found that the problem was far more frequent after the delivery of a baby than after an induced abortion (Brewer, 1977). The author suggests that psychological changes after childbirth are probably greater than after abortion and may be responsible for the higher incidence of psychosis after delivery of a baby.

Although some studies have described a higher incidence of psychological symptoms among younger women (Zolese and Blacker, 1992), a study specifically designed to evaluate this issue found that, following induced abortion, the scores for women as young as fourteen years equaled those for older women on several psychological scales (Pope, Adler, and Tschann, 2001). The same authors found an increase in positive emotions after (compared with before) abortion. It is also unclear whether having a previous child affects the chance of psychological disturbance, as different studies show conflicting results (Payne et al., 1976; Zolese and Blacker, 1992).

The main conclusion is that pregnancy termination does not have negative psychological consequences for women who make the decision with no external pressure. This was also the unanimous conclusion of a panel of experts assembled by the American Psychological Association to examine legal abortion in the United States (Adler, 1989). Although there have been anecdotal descriptions of severe depression and even psychosis many years after abortion (Butler, 1996), it is unclear whether these women would have suffered the same or even worse psychological disturbances if the abortions had not taken place (Handy, 1982; Dagg,1991).

The authors of a transnational review of this issue carried out in the

1970s concluded that the most common psychological consequence of abortion "was, by far, that of relief" (David et al, 1978, p. 3). Moreover, it is important to consider the psychological effects of denying abortion, as unwanted childbirth may cause severe consequences for both mother and child. A high risk of social and interpersonal difficulties has been described among children who are the product of unwanted pregnancies (Furstenberg, Brooks-Gunn, Chase-Lansdale, 1989; Dagg, 1991).

Social Consequences

Under many circumstances, induced abortion results in effects that compare positively with the effects of enduring unwanted pregnancy. Adolescent girls who have no children and who abort unwanted pregnancies tend to continue their studies, whereas those (like *Roberta*'s sister) who opt to continue their pregnancies are usually forced to discontinue their education (Bailey et al., 2001). In circumstances of poverty and lack of expectations, however, having a baby may have a more positive effect on self-esteem than choosing to abort (Bailey et al., 2001).

In contrast, in some African countries, complications from unsafe abortions, such as genital infection that leads to infertility or chronic pelvic pain, can make it difficult for women to perform the functions that society assigns them. In practice, this can mean that their role in society is downgraded and they end up marginalized from their communities. The resulting social consequences include family disruption and different forms of ostracism for the woman (Ladipo, 1989; Liskin, 1992).

Economic Consequences

A clean, safe abortion, performed in an appropriate facility, costs less than the average delivery, whereas the care of a woman with complications from an unsafe abortion can put a heavy economic burden on a health system. In many developing countries, complications from unsafe abortions consume a large proportion of available health care resources: hospital beds, surgical theater time, medical equipment, antibiotics, intravenous fluids, blood and blood products, disposable supplies, and specialized human resources (Fortney, 1981; Bugalho, 1995).

Chile was one of the first countries that studied this problem seriously and began to implement solutions. In the early 1960s, physicians in Chile's public health and obstetrics system documented the impact of abortion on health care. In 1963 approximately 20 percent of the country's obstetric beds were occupied by women with abortion complications, who represented 8 percent of all patients discharged from the nation's hospitals (Plaza and Briones, 1962). A decade or two later, as many as 30 percent of hospital beds allocated to obstetrical and gynecological care in Latin America were occupied by women with abortion complications (Viel, 1982).

It is important to note that the number of patients with abortion complications, calculated as a percentage of the total number of patients discharged from hospitals, is not a true indicator of the effect of abortion on health care resources. This is because each patient with abortion complications uses more staff time and more surgical, medical, and laboratory resources and requires longer hospitalization than the average hospitalized individual or any other obstetrical patient. An illustration of this phenomenon is that in 1993 in Maputo, Mozambique, the cost of treating a patient for complications resulting from an unsafe illegal abortion was nine times higher than the cost of performing a clean, in-hospital pregnancy termination and five times higher than the cost of delivery. Complications from unsafe abortions resulted in the use of one hundred times more antibiotics and sixteen times more blood transfusions, and in hospitalizations that were fifteen times longer than for women who underwent in-hospital pregnancy termination (Bugalho, 1995).

Although the problem in Latin American remains serious, the 1970s and 1980s saw the beginning of a wave of improvement in some Latin American countries, in parallel with increased access to contraceptive methods. The abortion scene in Sub-Saharan Africa today appears to be comparable to the scene in Latin America in the 1960s and 1970s.

Factors That Influence the Severity of the Consequences of Abortion

The technical and hygienic conditions under which an abortion is performed have the greatest effect on the severity of the complications, but the following factors are also relevant: the gestational age at which termination takes place, the length of time between the occurrence of a complication and access to a health facility, and the quality of health care received (Cates et al., 1977; Atrash et al., 1987).

These medical factors are affected by a society's legal and cultural attitude toward abortion and by the economic status of the woman who aborts. In countries where abortion is legal and is culturally accepted, the procedure can be performed safely in appropriate hospital facilities. In countries with restrictive laws and a negative public view of those who choose to abort and those who implement the abortions, the situation is reversed. These two major non-medical factors that influence the severity of the consequences of induced abortions will be discussed below

The Legal Status of Abortion and Access to Safe Abortions

The consequences of abortion for both women and society will depend on progress in the legal arena and increased access to safe abortion. Abortion-related mortality is generally highest in countries where abortion is legally restricted and reproductive health services are inadequate or nonexistent. In contrast, in countries where abortion is legal and services are adequate, no woman who opts to abort need put her health at risk (Sundström, 1996).

The best example of the effect of legal access to safe abortion and its prohibition comes from Romania. Until November 1965, when a liberal law was replaced with a totally restrictive law, the abortion-related maternal mortality rate was below 20 per 100,000 live births. Between 1966 and 1988, the non-abortion-related maternal mortality continued

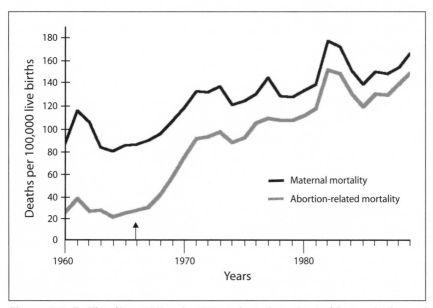

Figure 4.1 . The Effect of Romania's November 1965 anti-abortion law on the rate of abortion-related maternal mortality. Source: Stephenson et al., 1992; WHO, 1997.

to decline, but the abortion-related maternal mortality increased approximately eightfold, to almost 150 per 100,000 live births (Stephenson et al., 1992; WHO, 1997). The increase in the abortion-related maternal death rate was the price paid by Romanian women who rejected the government's pressure to force them to have more children than they wanted.

Access to legal abortion services depends as much on the attitude of health care providers and the organization of the health system as on the laws. Although low-income women have greater access to safe abortions in countries where they are legal than in counties where they are not, liberalization of abortion laws does not always guarantee that abortion services will be available. Zambia and India are two examples of countries where, because neither the health system nor the physicians are prepared to meet the demand, legality has little effect on access to safe abortion.

In India, the MTP Act legalized abortion in 1972. Since that time, although the number of reported MTP cases has been slowly increasing, it has remained relatively small. The number of institutions approved to provide MTP rose from 1,877 in 1976 to 7,121 in 1991, and the number of MTP cases increased from 25 between 1972 and 1973 to 632,526 between 1991 and 1992. It was estimated, however, that an additional 5 to 6 million abortions were performed in India every year, mostly in rural areas with inadequate facilities and unsafe conditions (Khan, Barge, and Philip, 1996).

Mohammad Ejazuddin Khan, Sandhya Barge, and George Philip (1996) concluded that even after twenty years of legalized abortion in India, services (particularly in rural areas) were inaccessible to the majority of women. Consequently, untrained practitioners, working in unhygienic conditions, performed 90 percent of the estimated 6.7 million induced abortions. More recent estimates show a rapid increase in the total number of abortions, including those that are legal, but the proportion of all abortions performed in unsafe conditions seems to have remained unchanged (Jain, 2001). Therefore, for the great majority of Indian women who voluntarily decide to terminate their pregnancies, legalized abortion has not decreased the risk to their health and their lives.

The situation is very similar in countries that have restrictive abortion laws but allow pregnancy termination in special cases, such as serious risk to the woman's life, rape, or severe fetal malformation. Frequently, women who fall into these categories do not have access to safe pregnancy termination and must resort to unsafe abortion. This is the case in most of Latin America and Africa, and also in some parts of Europe (Vilar, 2002).

Access to legal termination of pregnancy when a woman's life is at risk is at the discretion of the physicians, who must assess whether the severity of the condition justifies the abortion. Evaluations vary from doctor to doctor, according to individual religious beliefs and cultural values and according to their sensitivity toward the level of risk that each woman is prepared to run. More often than not, however, women's opinions are neither requested nor considered, leaving physicians as the sole decision makers in the process.

In the case of pregnancy that results from rape, proof of conception during rape is generally required for hospital administrators and physicians to approve a pregnancy termination. Although the laws of most countries do not specify the procedure, hospitals usually require a judicial order. Because this process frequently takes longer than human gestation, the law is, in practice, rarely applied (Pitanguy and Garbayo, 1995). Moreover, even women who manage to obtain a judicial order may be refused public hospital care by physicians who feel threatened by anti-abortion groups and fear religious condemnation.

Lack of access to safe abortions in public hospitals forces women of limited means who have the legal right to pregnancy termination to expose themselves to the risks of undergoing unsafe, unregulated abortions. Thus, the prevailing culture, the balance of political power between groups in favor of or against the criminalization of abortion, and the attitude of health care providers (particularly physicians) are important determining factors in the severity of the consequences of induced abortion on both women and society.

Socioeconomic Status

As we have noted, in most societies where abortion is legally restricted, women of means have access to clandestine but safe abortion. In contrast, women without these economic resources must resort to the services of nonprofessional abortionists whose dangerous and unhygienic methods have catastrophic consequences. There is much anecdotal evidence and media coverage of the various levels of sophistication at private, semi-clandestine abortion clinics, with safe and costly abortion available to women of means (Barros, Santa Cruz, and Sanches, 1997) but unavailable to those of limited means, who must risk the severe consequences of unsafe abortion (Bhuiya, Aziz, and Chowdhury, 2001). One study in Egypt, for example, found that the cost of a safe illegal abortion was up to two and a half times the country's average monthly per capita income, whereas the cost of an unsafe abortion was less than one U.S. dollar (Lane, Jok, and El-Mouelhy, 1998).

The correlation between the consequences of abortion and socio-economic status is also observed in some countries with liberal abortion laws. Between 1972 and 1982, mortality associated with the legal termination of pregnancy in the United States was about three times higher among African American women than among white women (Atrash et al., 1987). Race is a well-known indicator of socioeconomic status in the United States, even more so during the period of the study in question than today. In addition, since public health insurance (Medicaid) does not cover the costs of abortion in many states, low-income women sometimes reach the second trimester of pregnancy before they are able to pay for the procedure (Henshaw and Wallisch, 1984; Henshaw and Finer, 2003). Differences in quality of care and in access to legal abortion services are socioeconomic inequalities that prevail in both developed and developing countries.

5

Why Women Get Pregnant
When They Do Not Want To

The most common reason given for why women have unintended and unwanted pregnancies is that they lack information about and/or access to contraceptive methods (Henshaw, Singh, and Haas, 1999). This is undoubtedly true both for unmarried women and for married women who already have the children they want. This was the case with *Rosa* the peasant and *Maria*, the middle class woman, in the stories told in Chapter 1. Both became pregnant against their will because they lacked accurate information about how to prevent pregnancy or were unable to overcome the economic, cultural, or physical obstacles to the use of contraception.

However, it is appropriate to recognize other circumstances that often fail to be taken into consideration in discussions on why women abort. Another important cause of unwanted pregnancy, even in women who are educated and financially independent, is the woman's inability to exercise control over when and under what circumstances she will have sexual relations, as in the case of *Blanca* and *Cristina*, the two physicians in the stories in Chapter 1.

Sometimes, women get pregnant because they want to have a child, but then their situation changes. A woman may experience negative pressure from a social group, her partner may threaten to abandon her or may simply disappear, her employer may force her to decide between her job and having the baby, her school may not accept pregnant students, or her family may not provide her with the support she expected (see the story of *Luisa* in Chapter 1).

Clearly, the circumstances that lead a woman to find herself confronted with a pregnancy she cannot allow to continue are not limited to lack of access to or knowledge of contraception. If we are serious in our intention to reduce the number of abortions worldwide, we must consider each of the circumstances that can lead to unplanned or unwanted pregnancy.

Each of the circumstances leading to abortion merits a more detailed discussion to fully understand its significance and to be able to resolve the problems that lead women to place themselves at risk and undergo the hardships of pregnancy termination.

Lack of Knowledge about Contraceptive Methods

There is vast information, derived mostly from the Demographic and Health Surveys (DHS 2002) population-based studies, that use a single set of research criteria and are carried out globally, permitting comparison among countries. According to these surveys, a high proportion of women worldwide state that they have knowledge of at least one "modern," highly effective contraceptive method. The definition of *modern* includes hormonal methods, intrauterine devices, barrier methods (such as the diaphragm and the male or female condom), and male or female surgical sterilization.

The percentage of women who declared that they knew of at least one of these methods varied from under 50 percent in Chad; to between 60 and 70 percent in Mozambique, Mali, Guinea, and Madagascar; to close to 98 percent in Kenya, Zambia, Nepal, and the Philippines (DHS, 2002). The proportion of women who declared that they knew at least one modern contraceptive method reached virtually 100 percent not only in developed countries but also in some less developed countries such as Bangladesh, the Dominican Republic, and Brazil.

These studies also show significant differences within each country, according to the place of residence (urban or rural) and socioeconomic status. The number of years of schooling is the main factor that determines contraceptive knowledge. As a result, in virtually every less developed country, 98 percent or more of women who have a secondary education or higher declared that they were aware of at least one modern contraceptive method; this was true for only about 50 percent of women with no education in Cameroon, Madagascar, Mozambique, the Philippines, and Bolivia.

If we move from the knowledge of at least one method to information on specific contraceptives, the differences by educational level are even more dramatic. In Brazil, virtually all women at every level of society know at least one modern method. This high level of knowledge is attributed to almost universal exposure to television, with its direct and subliminal messages (Faria and Potter, 1999). Condoms have been the subject of mass media campaigns, as have the two most popular methods: female sterilization and pills. Nevertheless, the choices are much more limited for women with no education. Only 12 percent of Brazilian women without a formal education declared that they knew the diaphragm or other vaginal methods in 1996, 42 percent knew the IUD, and 45 percent declared that they knew male of sterilization. This contrasts with 90 percent, 98 percent, and 98 percent, respectively, for women with higher education.

As dramatic as they are, these quantitative differences do not tell the whole story. The first DHS question asked is "Which contraceptives do you know about?" Then each method that the interviewee fails to mention is named, and the interviewee says whether she knows it. This means that any woman who has heard of a method is included as "knowing about" the method. It may be that her "knowledge" is totally distorted or completely wrong. She may "know," for example, the following false information: that the IUD causes an abortion every month (as *Maria,* the working-class urban woman was told when she stopped using the pill) or that women who take the pill for too long become sterile. These are just some of the many false rumors that prevent women from using these methods. (Osis et al., 2003).

The few studies that have explored the accuracy of knowledge about contraceptive methods have shown discouraging results. A study showed that among women living in the most impoverished areas of Rio de Janeiro, 23 percent of those who used contraceptive pills were using them incorrectly (Costa et al., 1990). Similarly, other studies have shown that adolescents and women with little education who attempt to use periodic abstinence for fertility control do so without accurate knowledge of the menstrual cycle and the fertile period (Cumming, Cumming, and Kieren, 1991; Castaneda, Garcia, and Langer, 1996). A study among South African students found that 85 percent were not aware that a condom should be put on before the penis makes contact with the vagina (Peltzer, 2001). Inaccurate knowledge of proper condom use was also found in a national sample of secondary school students in the United States. About one-third of female students and two-fifths of male students who were sexually active and almost half of male and female students who were not sexually active were not aware of the importance of leaving a space in the tip of the condom. One-third of both groups believed wrongly that Vaseline could be used with condoms (Crosby and Yarber, 2001). Using a penile model, knowledge of correct condom use was assessed in a subsample of African-American adolescents. The study found that 75 percent did not squeeze the air from the tip when applying the condom (Crosby and Yarber, 2001). Adolescents in some less developed countries have an even greater disadvantage, since their basic knowledge of reproductive physiology can be so lacking that they are not even aware that girls can get pregnant the first time they have sexual intercourse (Oyediran, Ishola, and Adewuyi, 2002).

Inadequate knowledge about contraception can affect the ability of women to protect themselves against unintended pregnancies in at least two ways: (1) They may opt not to use a method, believing incorrectly that it may have a negative effect (for example, that IUDs cause cancer or that the pill causes infertility). (2) They may use it incorrectly, inadvertently exposing themselves to the risk of pregnancy as happened to *Maria* in the story reported earlier, who didn't know how important it was not to miss the first pills of the month. Again, the accuracy of information is affected by education level, increasing the social disadvantage of women who have less opportunity to attend school.

According to a national sample of adolescents in the United States, religious affiliation also negatively affected knowledge about condom use (Crosby and Yarber, 2001). In addition, distorted, sensationalist information disseminated by the media about certain methods has had a dramatic impact on the number of abortions in some developed countries. For example, after a reported increase in the risk of adverse vascular effects associated with the third-generation pill, an evaluation in Norway showed a dramatic decrease in the use of this method. This decrease, which was not immediately compensated by a proportional increase in the use of other contraceptive methods, caused a 36 percent rise in the abortion rate among fifteen- to twenty-four-year-old women (Skjeldestad, 1997).

Lack of Access to Contraceptive Methods

The most frequently used indicator of women's access to contraceptive methods is the *prevalence of use*—that is, the percentage of women of childbearing age who use contraception. The problem with this indicator, however, is that prevalence of use depends not only on access but also on *the demand for fertility regulation.* In societies where the fertility ideal is high, prevalence of use may be very low in spite of good access if what women desire is to have as many children as they can. For this reason, access to contraceptive methods is better evaluated through what has been called *unmet need* for contraceptives. *Unmet need* is defined as the proportion of women who do not want to get pregnant at that precise time or ever again and who are not using any contraceptive method.

Looking at the unmet need for contraceptive methods in less developed countries, it would appear that there are three stages: The first stage, in which the desire for fertility regulation is low and contraceptive use is therefore also very low, results in minimal unmet need. In the second stage, a higher percentage of women want to control their fertility, and access to contraceptive methods varies widely. This stage has the highest proportion of women with an unmet need for contraception. Finally, in the third stage, the percentage of women who want to control their fertility is highest, as is their access to modern contraceptive methods. At this stage, typical of developed countries, the proportion of women with an unmet need is low. This sequence of events is illustrated by the situation in different countries that are currently going through each of the three stages described above.: Chad, which has the lowest level of knowledge and use of modern contraceptive methods (43 percent and 1.2 percent, respectively), is in the first stage, with an unmet need of only 9.7 percent (DHS, 2002). Much higher percentages of unmet need, between 24 percent and 31 percent, are found in countries with an intermediate prevalence of use, examples of the second stage (Kenya, at 31.5 percent; Bolivia, at 25.2 percent; and Nepal, at 26 percent). The third stage is represented by developed and some developing countries, where the high demand is balanced by improved access to contraception and consequently the unmet need is low. Countries with a contraceptive prevalence (of modern methods) above 50 percent have an unmet need that is uniformly below 10 percent. The high unmet need for contraception in countries in the second stage may be one of the main factors that determine the prevalence of unsafe abortion. A study in Nepal found, for example, that for many women unsafe abortion was the only available method of fertility control (Tamang, Shrestha, and Sharma, 1999).

A superficial analysis may lead to the conclusion that countries in the first stage do not merit further attention. However, if we look at the data more carefully, the picture changes. The 9.7 percent of women with an unmet need in Chad may seem low, for example, but when we consider that only 1.2 percent of women were using a modern contraceptive method, it becomes apparent that nine out of every ten women who wished to prevent a pregnancy did not have access to contraception.

The first impression is that unmet need is equivalent to lack of availability of contraceptive methods. A more detailed observation reveals that other reasons contribute to unmet need: from lack of knowledge or lack of the resources needed to obtain contraceptives to lack of collaboration or opposition from partner and family to cultural pressure. These factors operate in different proportions in different environments, but whatever the reason for the unmet need, it will be closely associated with unwanted pregnancy and consequently with abortion.

As noted in Chapter 3, the highest abortion rates have been observed in countries in eastern and central Europe that belonged to the former Soviet Union. Contraceptive prevalence was low because only high-dose contraceptive pills associated with more side effects were available, the quality of condoms and IUDs was poor, and there were legal restrictions to surgical sterilization. In addition, because the public supply of contraceptive methods was unreliable, women were forced to control their fertility through abortion, the only easily accessible option (David, 1982; Popov, 1991).

The situation was similar in two of the developing countries with the highest abortion rates, Cuba and Vietnam (Hardy et al., 1990; Alvarez, 1992; Goodkind, 1994), which were also under strong Soviet influence until the late 1980s and remained relatively isolated in subsequent years. On the one hand, inadequate services and irregular supplies discouraged contraception, while on the other hand menstrual regulation and abortion were easily available.

Most Latin American countries that experienced a high birth rate until the 1960s began to see a decline in fertility in the following ten to twenty years, with a rapid reduction in the ideal family size. Because contraceptive methods were not easily available, the population turned to abortion, which reached an alarmingly high rate in some countries. The slow increase in the availability of contraceptive methods appeared to follow a curve parallel to the increase in the desire for smaller families, which prevented the expected reduction in abortion. Exceptions were the few countries with superior public health services that became involved in the widespread provision of various contraceptive methods. Easy access led to a rapid increase in use, which was followed by a reduction in the number of induced abortions (Maine, 1981; Viel, 1985; Barzelatto, 1986).

In conclusion, it seems clear that a large proportion of abortions occur as a result of a lack of access to contraceptive methods or accurate knowledge about their use.

Failure of Contraceptive Methods

Even the correct use of contraceptives does not guarantee that a woman will not become pregnant. In fact, in some studies more than half of abortions occurred among women who were using a contraceptive method when they became pregnant (Alvarez et al., 1999; Sparrow, 1999). Methods fail (1) because they are not infallible or (2) because they are used improperly. Traditional methods, such as periodic abstinence and coitus interruptus, have a high failure rate that is partially the result of the intrinsic ineffectiveness of the methods, but mostly the result of improper use (WHO, 1981; Indian Council of Medical Research, 1996).

Similarly, although the birth control pill's effectiveness is close to 100 percent in controlled clinical studies, the failure rates observed in population-based studies are closer to 8 percent per year of use (Potter, 1996; Trussell, 1998). Several studies have shown that many pill users have not been instructed on proper use, frequently forget to take it, or delay the initiation of a new cycle if they will be separated from their partner for a few days. Most pill users are unaware that the chances of failure greatly increase if the pill-free interval is prolonged for even a few days.

Of course, there are virtually no user failures for methods that do not depend on user compliance, such as intrauterine devices and implants. Some of the newer versions of these methods, such as the Copper T-380 and progestin-releasing IUDs and implants, are among the most effective contraceptives available (Chi, 1991; Croxatto and Makarainen, 1998; Mishell, 1998). Since these characteristics make them highly effective in reducing unwanted pregnancies and abortions, they should be included among contraceptive methods available to women. Equally important is that women should know about these methods and take them into consideration when choosing which contraceptive method they will use.

Lack of Control in Sexual Relationships

Often women have the knowledge about and access to contraceptive methods but do not have control over their use every time they have sexual relations. In addition, they may not be using a method because they are not having sexual relations and are then unexpectedly forced to have sex without the means or the time to protect themselves. Far from being a rare event, sex against a woman's will is a rather common occurrence. The first problem is to establish the definition of imposed sex. It ranges from armed physical aggression through the cultural imposition of male "rights" over a woman's body. Most studies are limited to the occurrence of rape, which is defined as imposed sexual intercourse using force or the threat of force. Their data do not include sexual coercion in exchange for obtaining or maintaining a job, passing an exam, or satisfying other personal needs. More subtle forms of imposition include a woman's sense of obligation to engage in sex in exchange for favors received or in deference to a stable, established relationship that may or may not involve marriage.

Studies on sexual violence show a prevalence that varies from less than 10 percent to about 40 percent of women of childbearing age (Heise, Pitanguy, and Germain, 1994; Golding, Wilsnack, and Learman, 1998). The differences in prevalence appear to be related as much to social distinctions between populations as to the various methods used to obtain the information and the different definitions of sexual violence. According to the United Nations, the definition of *gender-based violence* includes threatening and coercion (United Nations, 1993), but many studies consider only direct physical imposition as sexual violence. More commonly, women are culturally conditioned to put satisfying the sexual desires of a partner or husband above their own wishes and above the risk of unwanted pregnancy (Maforah, Wood, and Jewkes, 1997; Zheng et al., 2001).

Rape, although prevalent, is not often associated with unwanted pregnancy. Far more relevant are the more subtle cultural imposition of unwanted sex and the inability to make use of available protection during desired sex (Maforah, Wood, and Jewkes, 1997; Zheng et al., 2001).

In a study carried out in one of the most developed regions of Brazil, 30 percent of the women interviewed reported having experienced physical imposition of sex or sexual coercion. An additional 32 percent of women admitted having had sex against their will because they felt obliged to comply with their partner's desire (Faúndes et al., 2000). Women who have knowledge about and access to a diaphragm or a condom or who intend to use periodic abstinence may not feel sufficiently empowered to refuse sex when they lack such protection, as in the case study of *Cristina*, the well-to-do physician, in Chapter 1.

The importance of gender power imbalance and negotiation around condom use that has been highlighted by studies related to the risk of acquiring AIDS may also apply to the risk of unwanted pregnancy (Maxwell and Boyle, 1995; Bajos and Marquet, 2000). A study among adolescent girls in the United States showed that a substantial proportion believed that boys who had invested time or money in entertaining their female partners had the right to have sex with them. The proportion was even higher among male adolescents in the United States and represented an overwhelming majority among adolescents in a study in South Africa (Jewkes et. al., 2001).

Most studies also show that both adolescent and adult males believe that protection against pregnancy is solely the responsibility of the woman (Pachauri, 2001). A study in India among women who requested legal termination of pregnancy found that one-third of unwanted pregnancies could be attributed to the husband's unwillingness to use contraception or improper or irregular condom use (Banerjee et al., 2001). Clearly—particularly among adolescents, in whom reduction of the abortion rate has been most difficult to achieve—male dominance in the decision to have sex and the lack of male responsibility for the use of contraception contribute to the occurrence of unintended pregnancy (McCauley and Salter, 1995; Maforah, Wood, and Jewkes, 1997; Sparrow, 1999).

As long as women are not empowered to control when and under what conditions they will have sex, they will be at risk for unwanted pregnancy. Thus, the prevalent pattern of gender power imbalance, which is more marked in less developed countries, is another condition that maintains the high incidence of induced abortion regardless of women's knowledge and access to contraceptive methods.

6

When Is a Pregnancy So Unwanted That It Ends in Abortion?

No woman takes pleasure in having an abortion. For some women abortion may cause little stress, but for the majority of women, it is a very disturbing experience that they would much prefer to avoid (Barros, Santa Cruz, and Sanches, 1997). "Abortion is a horrendous ordeal"; "People who have not had to go through the trauma of abortion would do well not to comment on the subject"; "I found myself in this unfortunate position [of choosing to abort]" were comments made by women who defended the availability of the abortion pill (mifespristone) during a recent public debate in the United Kingdom (Daily Record Debate, 2002). Pregnancy has to be really very unwanted to lead a woman to undergo an abortion. In fact, many women who were interviewed following a voluntary termination of pregnancy commented that they had opposed abortion before they found themselves facing the choice to abort (Bengtsson and Wahlberg, 1991).

Women in both developed and developing countries share this view. A study in Cuba, for example, where abortion is highly prevalent, showed that 78 percent of women who had had a voluntary pregnancy termination remained opposed to or were ambivalent about abortion (Alvarez et al., 1999). The authors commented that "frank approval of this approach to fertility regulation is minimal . . . in contrast with their attitude towards contraception, which is highly positive" (Alvarez et al., 1999, p. 129). Similarly, a study in Brazil found that a significant proportion of women who had had induced abortions continued to oppose abortion under any circumstance (Osis et al., 1994). These studies confirm, therefore, that abortion is a decision that women do not take lightly and their motives have to be very strong.

Studies show that the many reasons for deciding to terminate preg-

nancy are fairly constant worldwide, although the prevalence of one reason or another may vary from one society to another. The most common
reasons can be grouped as follows: the absence of the father, financial
constraints, the inability to provide good parenting or interference with
life prospects, conflict with prevailing social norms, health concerns, and
lack of social support.

The Absence of the Father

Nelly was single, the twenty-one-year-old daughter of a peasant
woman and an unknown father. She had migrated to the big city and
was employed as a maid for a middle-class family. She worked as
many as fourteen hours a day, Monday through Saturday, with time
off only on Sundays and occasionally on Saturday nights. In her free
time, she would get together with her boyfriend, who had promised
to marry her as soon as he could find a better job. When Nelly
became pregnant, however, no sooner had he heard the news than he
disappeared. Even though Nelly had had a stepfather since she was
only three, she had suffered the cruel words of her schoolmates and
neighbors about the absence of her biological father. Determined not
to have a child of hers suffer the same humiliation, she decided to
abort.

This story illustrates how heavily the absence of a partner who would
assume his role as father can weigh on the decision to abort. This circumstance is prevalent not only among young, unmarried women but also
among older women, who may have been abandoned by a partner or who
may be in an unstable partnership (Torres and Forrest, 1988; Barnett,
Freudenberg, and Wille, 1992; Justesen, Kapiga, and van Asten, 1992;
Skjeldestad, 1994; Törnbom et al., 1994; Gupte, Bandewar, and Pisal,
1997; Törnbom and Möller, 1999). It appears that the lack of a functional
family unit is a strong motivation to abort (Kero et al., 1999).

Financial Constraints

Flora was a twenty-eight-year-old wife and mother. She had two
children, ages two and seven. The seven-year-old had been diagnosed
with poliomyelitis, had been hospitalized for more than a month, and
would now require expensive rehabilitation therapy to recover full

use of his legs. In the midst of her child's diagnosis and illness, Flora had lost track of the schedule she had been following in the rhythm method, and she had become pregnant. Her husband's income was barely enough to feed their family of four, and now it was being stretched to pay for her older son's physiotherapy. Convinced that they simply could not afford another child, she decided to abort.

Especially, but not exclusively, in developing countries, the lack of financial resources to support a future child or sufficiently care for existing children is frequently expressed (Elu, 1999). In fact, this financial insecurity is no more frequent in the poorest sectors than it is among the middle classes (Costa et al., 1990). Expectations for their children's future are of key importance, as we saw in the case study of *Maria*, the wife of a bank employee (see Chapter 1). This may be more common in countries that have suffered severe economic constraints after a period of relatively comfortable socioeconomic conditions, such as countries of the ex-Soviet Union, where lack of resources to raise another child is frequently alleged as a reason for aborting (Dougherty, 2001).

The Inability to Provide Good Parenting/ Interference with Life Prospects

Sometimes it is not only the inability to provide material goods that motivates a woman to abort but also the perception that she will be unable to provide good parenting. Especially among adolescents, the feeling that they lack the maturity or preparation for motherhood is often expressed. Among unmarried teenagers in developed countries and among the educated elite in developing countries, the belief that pregnancy and motherhood would interfere with educational and employment life prospects is a common reason for aborting (Torres and Forrest, 1988; Törnbom et al., 1994). A study at a Brazilian university showed that 74 percent of students twenty-four years of age and under who became pregnant had abortions, whereas only 36 percent of female staff members in the same age group aborted their pregnancies (Hardy, Rebello, and Faúndes, 1993). Further analysis of qualitative aspects of the same study showed that the primary reason for aborting was inability to care for or educate the child (Costa et al., 1995). Although age is an important factor in feeling unprepared to be a mother, a woman's expectations of the life achievements she must fulfill before she becomes a mother appear to be equally important.

Countries that maintain high fertility offer another expression of limited ability to provide good parenting as a reason for abortion. Egyptian women with numerous children reported having reached the limit of their capacity to care for their children as a reason for not wanting to continue to give birth (Huntington, Nawar, and Abdel-Hady, 1997). In other words, even women whose ideal is to be the mother of many children realize that they cannot provide good mothering care to an unlimited number of offspring.

Conflict with Prevailing Social Norms

A September 15, 2002, *Boston Globe* article tells the story of two women in northern Nigeria who were condemned to death by stoning for the crime of adultery (Doran, 2002). The women, both widows, had each given birth to a baby, proof of their illicit sexual relationships. Women who live in societies with such rigorous restrictions on extramarital sexual activity will often choose to abort a pregnancy that does not comply with the accepted norms.

The situation is not very different in many Western societies, with restrictive social norms of their own. Transgressors do not risk being sentenced to death by stoning, but they risk other forms of segregation that can destroy their social lives. In Latin America extramarital childbirth may be more socially acceptable among the lower-income population than among middle- or upper-class families. When there is no hope of arranging a marriage before a pregnancy becomes evident, the only way to preserve both the family's honor and the social future of the pregnant woman is to abort.

Health Concerns

Abortions for health reasons are most prevalent in impoverished countries (Oodit and Bhowon, 1999). This can be explained, in part, because other reasons for abortion occur less frequently in these countries, but also because in societies that place great value on high fertility, only a threat to life can justify the decision to abort as illustrated by the story of *Rosa*, the peasant mother of six, described in Chapter 1. For many women, the motivation to preserve their own lives is the risk to their children's well-being if they become motherless.

Lack of Social Support

> *Gabriela*—twenty-two years old, single, and the mother of a four-year-old son being cared for by her mother—was working in a factory for a paltry salary and living in her parents' home. When her father found out that she was pregnant again, he kicked her out of the house. Her boyfriend vanished, and she ended up moving in with a friend who was willing to accept Gabriela but not a baby into her home. Gabriela saw no solution but to abort.

> *Marisol* worked as a maid for a relatively wealthy family. When her boss learned that she was pregnant, he told her that she would have to leave. Marisol's job as a maid provided her with not only a salary but also food and lodging. She had no one else to turn to. The only way for her to survive was to abort.

These two stories illustrate the circumstances of women who cannot choose to have their babies because they lack the support they need from their families or their employers.

Except in some of the most highly developed countries, women worldwide are left alone to reproduce with very little support from society. Although, in theory, legislation in most countries protects women during pregnancy, labor, and lactation, the laws are usually poorly written and are rarely effective. In most cases, pregnant women struggle to maintain an income and spend long hours queuing to obtain basic, and sometimes inadequate, prenatal and delivery care. After delivery, they rarely find child care facilities close enough to their place of employment to allow them to breastfeed and keep their jobs. Confronted with this harsh reality, in which social support is almost totally absent, those who do not have a supportive partner or an understanding family see no alternative but to abort as illustrated by the case of young *Luisa*, described in Chapter 1.

In all the situations we have described, the decision not to give birth, far from being selfish, showed a sense of responsibility, the desire to prevent a situation in which a child would be born into an environment unconducive to healthy development. Recent reports of an increase in the incidence of dead newborn babies left in the streets of Moscow show the dramatic consequences of lack of access to abortion among women who live in what they believe to be conditions that are inadequate for the care of their children (Stephen, 2002). This trend smacks of a return to the Middle Ages, when abortion was so risky that women were forced to turn to infanticide (see the discussion in Chapter 8).

The general conclusion is that in most cases, the decision to abort is an expression of each woman's sense of concern about the responsibilities of motherhood or about the protection of her future or the future of her existing family.

PART II
Values

7
Conflicting Values Encountered by Health Professionals

When I (AF) was a medical intern, in the 1950s, I worked in the emergency department of a hospital in Chile. My schedule was Monday through Saturday from 6:30 to 9:00 p.m., in addition to one night in six and one full Sunday in six. Because the shift chief knew that I had already decided to specialize in obstetrics and gynecology, soon after my internship began, I was sent to work in the "curettage" room, where incomplete abortions were treated. There were so many that, I often spent the whole two and a half hours of my shift doing nothing but curettage, particularly on Friday and Saturday evenings.

At the time, the prevailing culture in medicine was to treat women who had abortions as criminals. Members of the public health system staff felt that they had the authority to accuse, judge, and condemn every woman with abortion complications and make them all suffer the pain of the curettage without anesthesia of any kind. If a woman dared to complain, she was verbally abused: She had to pay for yielding to the pleasures of sex without assuming the responsibility of motherhood. The presumption was that (1) she had wanted to have sex, (2) she had enjoyed it, (3) she had not prevented the pregnancy because she was irresponsible, and (4) her reasons for not wanting to continue the pregnancy were selfish. At first I bought into this line of thought, but as I began to listen to the women's stories, it become increasingly clear that in almost every case, some or all of of the four presumptions listed above were incorrect.

My initial condemnation of these women shifted to understanding and compassion. I rebelled against a society that pushed women into a situation where they saw no other choice but to submit to the risk and pain of an unsafe abortion. I also came to realize that the abortion epidemic that was rapidly growing in the country at the time was just the sum of numerous examples of "exceptional circumstances" and that each woman had a valid justification for deciding to terminate her pregnancy.

At the same time, I was under the illusion that it would be possible to prevent abortions if women knew about and had access to effective contraceptive methods. It took some time and accumulated experience to realize that some abortions will always occur.

Health Professionals and the Value of Life

For health care providers, saving lives is the primary goal, and for those who care for a pregnant woman, this goal includes both the life of the potential mother and that of her offspring. It is with this perspective in mind that we consider the reasons and circumstances under which health care providers reach the decision to accept or reject a woman's request to terminate a pregnancy.

Most young students are motivated to enter medical school by the desire to help people by means of curing diseases and saving lives. Many of them have witnessed the skillful and timely intervention of a physician who alleviated the suffering of a friend or relative. Therefore, right from the very beginning of a career in medicine, the main motivation of medical students is to acquire the power to save lives through the knowledge and experience gained during the training process.

When the time comes to choose a specialty, those who choose obstetrics are typically motivated by the ability to contribute to the process of bringing new life into the world. The miracle of birth is the most positive experience any person can have, in contrast to the other extreme in a physician's duties, that of helping a patient to die **without** pain and with the greatest possible dignity

Obstetricians and the Fetus

Obstetrics is an extremely rewarding medical specialty, and those who practice it feel most satisfied by the birth of a healthy infant. In difficult cases, particularly if the baby's life was at considerable risk during labor and delivery, obstetricians are rewarded with the legitimate pride of having been instrumental in "giving" the mother a healthy child. This feeling of power and gratification is reinforced by the appreciation that mothers often express to their obstetricians weeks, months, or even years later.

The obstetrician's work is as dedicated to the health and life of the fetus as it is to the health and life of the woman in his or her care. From the first prenatal visit, the obstetrician's attentions are focused as much on verifying the normalcy of fetal development as on ensuring the health and well-being of the potential mother as she goes through the bodily changes caused by the progression of her pregnancy.

Women who want to have a baby entrust the health of their future child, as well as their own health, to their physician, often showing more concern for their offspring than for themselves. Typically, the obstetrician becomes as attached to the fetus as to his or her pregnant patient. It is necessary to understand this subculture of obstetrical practice in order to grasp how traumatic the idea of abortion can be for an obstetrician.

Medical Technology and the Presence of the Fetus

During the initial weeks, pregnancy is fundamentally an abstraction, marked by discomforts and annoyances: feelings of bloating, nausea, and vomiting; intolerance of odors and certain foods; frequent urination; and painful breasts. These less than pleasant changes are the indications that the woman's body is under the influence of something new. Until recently, the perception of fetal movement was the first direct indication that a new person was developing within a woman. From that moment on, the emotional mother/child attachment grows.

With the introduction of sonar equipment, which has enabled early identification of the fetus's heartbeats, this situation began to change. Sonar sends a sound wave toward the fetus's heart, transforms the movements of the beating heart into a sound, and sends it back in the form of another sound wave. In this way, the fetal heartbeats can be "heard" before they are audible through a stethoscope and several weeks before fetal movements are perceived.

All that changed again with the development of ultrasonography, which has become increasingly efficient at "viewing" the growth and development of the embryo and fetus inside the womb. At the present time, with ultrasound technology, the developing embryo is "visible" and photographable as early as six weeks after the woman's last menstruation or two weeks after her missed period. "Viewing" the embryo at this stage—even though it is no more than a mass of cells within the embryonic sac, with no resemblance to a human form and no distinction from the embryo of any other mammal (Morowitz and Trefil, 1992)—can have a profound psychological effect. Of course, the emotional impact increases even further once the shape of the fetus can be distinguished.

The opportunity to observe the ultrasonic images of the early embryo and of the fetus has become one of the main motivations for couples to seek prenatal care. These photographic images have become a valued part of the family photo album in many cases. This new "visibility" of the embryo and fetus has converted what was once an abstraction into a new reality.

Technology and the Acceptance of Abortion

The "visibility" of the embryo through ultrasound technology has changed the subjective value that the embryo has for the woman, for the doctor, for the family, and for society. As long as the embryo/fetus was not visible, it remained merely a "missed period"; even if a woman knew she was pregnant, getting the uterine blood to flow again was not the same for many women as having an abortion (Osis et al., 1996).

For the physician, as long as the pregnancy represented just a change in the woman's body, abortion was merely a restoration of her previous condition, with only minor attention paid to the removed contents of the uterus. The physical visualization of the embryo by ultrasound increased the focus on what was being removed for the sake of the woman's physical, psychological, or social well-being.

The difference between the more abstract concept of terminating a "pregnancy," which is just a change in the woman's body, and the more concrete removal of an embryo that can be seen may appear to some as purely academic. For many physicians, however, visualization of the embryo makes a great difference and severely affects their capacity to accept abortion as the best solution in many circumstances in a woman's life. The pro-life movement has understood the power of the image of the developing embryo and, by attributing earlier gestational age to fetuses already in later development, has used and abused it. The misuse of such images is no justification, however, for ignoring the power of the "objectification" of the embryo, which ultrasound technology has brought to the abortion debate. The impact of this technology on the obstetrician/gynecologist, who must perform the abortion is a fact that must be considered in order to understand their attitude and behavior when confronted with a woman seeking an abortion.

Other technological developments have had the opposite effect on physicians. For those who have to evacuate the uterus, there is a big difference between D & C and vacuum aspiration of the uterine contents. During D & C, as soon as fetal parts can be distinguished (at about eight weeks of gestation) (Lumley, 1980), the physician can see those parts being removed by the curette. Vacuum aspiration, in contrast, allows physicians to remove fetal parts without actually seeing them, which makes a great difference in the impact abortion has on the practitioner.

Pharmacological means of early pregnancy termination further facilitate the procedure by eliminating the physical act of removing the embryo or fetus from the woman's uterus. Although the ultimate objective and result are exactly the same, it is always easier for the physician to accept and approve the woman's decision to terminate a pregnancy when he or she does not have to be directly involved in the action that results from that decision.. Pharmacological pregnancy termination places the physician several steps away from the role he or she has to play in a D & C, and that distance makes a very important psychological difference.

Obstetricians and Unwanted Pregnancies

For many obstetricians, interaction with pregnant women who do not want to be mothers is rare and sporadic. In developing countries, where abortion is legally restricted, people with no financial means, who constitute the great majority, know very well that if they want to abort an unintended and unwanted pregnancy, they can expect no help from the public health service. Because abortion services are completely separate from other obstetrical practices in the United States, most U.S. specialists have no contact with women who do not wish to continue their pregnancies but only with women who want to have a child.

As a result, in many countries—particularly where abortion is legally restricted—the majority of women who have unwanted pregnancies are all but invisible to the vast majority of obstetricians. The only interaction that many specialists have with unwanted pregnancies is limited to those women who have complications from illegal, unsafe, backdoor abortions. Alarmed and moved by the severe health consequences of unsafe abortion, many physicians initially react by condemning rather than understanding. The reaction is similar to that of physicians who treat a person who has suffered the consequences of an overdose of illegal drugs. They fall into the trap of viewing both types of patients as wrongdoers.

The circumstances that lead a woman to decide to have an abortion are seldom discussed and rarely understood. No sympathy is forthcoming; instead, condemnation and disapproval is the normal attitude of health professionals treating women with abortion complications. Influenced by their far more common experience with women who want to have a baby and who express their joy at the impending birth of their child, obstetricians tend to place themselves in opposition to women who abort and in favor of the fetus. It is far easier and more comfortable to condemn than to try to understand the motives of these women. It is only natural that those who chose obstetrics because of the positive feeling that giving birth creates in the mother, the family and in the practicing physician, do not feel comfortable with abortion and easily reject the idea of terminating a pregnancy with the inevitable loss of the fetus.

Cultural Pressures

The situation is even worse in countries where abortion is legally restricted and backdoor abortions are frequently connected to other illegal activities. In these cases, physicians who perform abortions usually have to do so through a network of police corruption and judicial bribery, which is usually associated with the cover-up of prostitution, drug trafficking, and other illegal activities.

There are a few examples of altruistic physicians who dedicate their lives to providing safe abortions in countries with severe legal restrictions to abortion. Apart from these exceptional cases, physicians in these countries who perform illegal abortions for profit can become very rich, but they tend to be excluded, as corrupt, from the elite circles of the medical establishment. They are viewed as having been corrupted by the money they earn since the high cost of their services is not justified by the medical intervention they perform but by the illegal, clandestine nature of the procedure. In such an environment, being an "abortionist" leads to a physician acquiring a bad reputation, and many women who use their services feel exploited and have no great respect for them. Ironically, however, abortionists are protected by the knowledge that their services may be needed at any time. Not infrequently, the most severe guardians of medical moral principles, publicly opposed to abortion, have requested the services of a despicable "abortionist" in the case of a relative or a friend "with a very personal problem due to very exceptional circumstances."

Physicians often position themselves against the practice of abortion because they do not want to break the law, the ethical dictates of the medical establishment, or the moral sanctions of their society's prevailing religion. Physicians are particularly sensitive to remaining within the law in their practice. The idea of being called to testify, being positioned before a judge as a defendant, terrifies most of us. Being submitted to the ethical judgment of the corresponding medical association is equally frightening, more so considering that such associations frequently have the power to temporarily or permanently suspend a physician's right to practice medicine.

Public Condemnation and Private Acceptance

The public condemnation of abortion in general does not prevent understanding and even the tacit and private approval of abortion under the "very personal and exceptional circumstances" of a relative, a friend or even a client.

A highly respected colleague and prestigious physician, who was a strict practicing member of the Catholic Church, had participated in several public debates with me (AF) on the subject of abortion. He argued that abortion was a sin and akin to homicide and that there were no circumstances under which this crime could be justified. We never managed to reach any agreement on the subject, yet we respected each other's opposing views given the transparent sincerity of our respective positions.   One night I received a telephone call from this colleague. His fifteen-year-old daughter had been at a party, where—after becoming inadvertently intoxicated on the sweet mixed drinks that she was served—she had been gang-raped by a group of boys. Now she was pregnant, and there was no way of knowing the identity of the "father" of her future child, therefore no possibility of an arranged marriage. My colleague was devastated. Above all, he wanted to protect his daughter from the shame. If her story came out, as it would if her pregnancy were allowed to continue, she would have no future, no hope of a "normal" family, no chance of happiness. Since his daughter's period was only two weeks late, and considering the extreme circumstances, my colleague thought that an early pregnancy termination was completely justified under these exceptional circumstances. Naturally, I agreed to help him arrange a safe abortion. The problem was solved, but from that day on my colleague steered clear of debates on abortion.

Although this story has particular idiosyncrasies, it serves to illustrate how even the strongest conviction in the abstract can dramatically change when the situation becomes personal.

Physicians' anti-abortion convictions can be shaken by experiences with not only relatives and friends but also clients. Obstetricians typically have clients who have been in their care for many years—through one, two, or even more pregnancies and deliveries. One day, one of these clients, who has placed all her trust in her doctor, may come to him or her with an unwanted pregnancy that she cannot possibly allow to go on. The initial reaction of the physician will usually be to try to convince the client that she should continue her pregnancy, and often he or she will succeed. If, however, the patient is not convinced and offers further personal reasons that make continuing the pregnancy unacceptable, her longtime physician will generally listen, try to understand her circumstances, and finally support her option to abort "in that particular case."

In spite of this support, the doctor generally declares that he/she does not perform abortions (Gonzalez and Salinas, 2000; Ramos et al., 2001). However, in most cases, the physician will help by giving the patient the address of a colleague who earns his living performing safe abortions (Faúndes et al., 2004). Most doctors will suggest that after the abortion has been carried out, the client should return to him or her to check that the abortion has not had any negative effect on the patient's health.

With the recent introduction of pharmacological abortion, some doctors who "do not do abortions" as a matter of principle are willing to instruct the patient on the use of misoprostol to induce an abortion. (Misoprostol, which has other medical uses, is far more accessible in the developing world than mifepristone, also known as RU 486 or the "abortion pill.") Doctors who accept the use of medical abortion, however, may continue to publicly condemn both women who have abortions and the physicians who help them.

From Accepting the Exception to Understanding the Rule

Few gynecologists have had the kind of experience described at the beginning of this chapter that in such a short time gave one of the authors (AF) the opportunity to listen to so many women who had had induced abortions. For most physicians it takes years to accumulate this kind of experience. Regardless of the time frame, however, many of us have followed the same path from initial condemnation to listening, to feeling perplexed and ambivalent, and finally to understanding that condemnation of women who abort is unjustified and futile. As we will see, the solution to the problem of abortion is very different and does not involve condemnation (McKay, Rogo, and Dixon, 2001).

Of course, not all obstetricians/gynecologists have followed this path. For many, the defense of the fetus remains their first priority and they maintain a position, at least in public, of strict condemnation of abortion under all or most circumstances. Even among these physicians, however, most of those who have an obstetrical/gynecological practice have on some occasions accepted that the circumstances of a particular patient who has decided to abort merit their understanding and compassion. Nevertheless, the gap is wide between private acceptance in "very exceptional cases" and public recognition of abortion as a personal and social problem that is not solved by criminalizing women who abort.

In a study carried out in Brazil in which forty-three hundred obstetricians / gynecologists responded to a questionnaire about abortion, 40 percent said that they had helped a client who had sought their advice regarding an absolutely unwanted pregnancy to obtain an abortion. Help consisted of referring the patient to an abortionist who would perform the procedure under the safest possible conditions; only a small minority had performed these abortions themselves. The percentage increased to 48 percent when the client was a family member. Furthermore, almost 80 percent of the unwanted pregnancies that occurred in female physicians themselves or in the partners of male physicians had ended in abortion (Faúndes et al., 2004). We believe that this is clear evidence that our capacity to understand and accept the circumstances of women who wish to abort an unwanted pregnancy increases progressively as we get closer to the problem.

Because they are faced with conflicting professional and moral values, health professionals in general and obstetricians and gynecologists in particular are frequently ambivalent about the problem of abortion. Although many refuse to perform abortions or even to support them publicly, most will accept, however, that abortions are morally justified under certain circumstances. The fundamental issue is that the perspective of gynecologists/obstetricians is unique for at least two reasons: (1) Their professional motivation and daily practice tends to center on the protection of the fetus. (2) They are the persons who actually perform the abortions, with all the associated legal, social, and psychological implications.

8

Religious Values

Most people in the world affiliate themselves with one religion or another, and their religious affiliation influences their thinking and actions. In fact, all people are influenced by the predominant religious values of the society in which they live, because these values are part of their culture. In some Muslim countries, the laws of Islam have been adopted as secular laws. In the past century or so, abortion has become a target for some religions, and some religious leaders have become key figures in the public debate on the subject. Consequently, an analysis of the values of (at least) the principal religions of the world as they relate to abortion is essential to any discussion of the issue.

We dedicate here a significant amount of the discussion to the Christian faiths, some of which (particularly the Catholic Church) have participated vocally in national and international debates on abortion policies. We, the authors of this book, have personally witnessed the important political role that the Catholic Church has played in abortion legislation in the Americas. Islamic perspectives have also figured prominently in the international abortion debate, mostly in the United Nations. We have omitted innumerable other traditions, particularly indigenous systems of belief, not only because of their diversity and comparatively smaller number of followers but also because they have played a negligible role in national or international policy discussions.

The task of describing the views of a particular faith on abortion or any other specific issue is a difficult one, because in no religion other than the Catholic Church is there a central authority that can act as the official voice of the faith. Moreover, throughout history, religious views on specific issues, including abortion, have changed, and the views of leaders within a particular faith have rarely been unanimous at any given point in time. At best, we can describe the views of the main schools of thought within a religion or the predominant views at a certain time in history. Even within the Catholic religion, the Pope's views—unless they are declared to be dogmas (a very rare occurrence that does not apply to abortion)—are open to question and change.

The sacred texts of the various religions are not specific enough to provide answers to most contemporary moral questions. Thus, the interpretation and application of all religious traditions to specific moral problems such as abortion have changed throughout history according to varying circumstances and the evolution of knowledge.*

The Historical Context of Christian Perspectives (Gudorf, 2003)

In order to understand Christian values and to put them in their proper perspective, it is necessary to look back into history. Contraception, abortion, and infanticide preceded Christianity. It may be a surprise to many that, in Europe as in the rest of the world, infanticide was used as a solution for unwanted pregnancy far more often than abortion. Infanticide was practiced throughout the Roman Empire, but Romans considered it to be barbarian and replaced it with abandonment as the preferred method.

Infanticide (frequently disguised as stillbirth) or abandonment were used because contraceptive methods were ineffective and abortion carried very high health risks, including extremely high mortality, for women. (An additional perceived advantage at the time was that infanticide or abandonment allowed for sex selection.) The extremely high mortality rate associated with abortion made it the last recourse of "the most desperate women," including "unmarried women, prostitutes, and adulteresses, all of whom faced the loss of their social place" by carrying their pregnancies to term. The association of abortion with such

---

*Compiling a brief review of religious values and abortion is a difficult challenge. We have the disadvantage and perhaps advantage of not being theologians. Therefore, as we have done throughout this book, we have relied on our life experiences. Both of us have seen the importance of religious values in abortion decisions and policies in our professional practices and in international activities, and José Barzelatto is one of the contributing authors of a book reviewing contraception and abortion in world religions (Barzelatto, J. and Dawson, E., 2003). To support our views, we have referred extensively to selected chapters of this book written by prominent theologians of various religions and to other important texts on the subject. When our main arguments are taken from one of these works, we have referenced the citation following the corresponding subhead.

social transgressions contributed to "stigmatize abortion as immoral in the minds of many" (Gudorf, 1998, p. 3). Today, as we have seen, the great majority of women who resort to abortion are in stable relationships and have quite different reasons for not wanting to continue their pregnancies.

As a result of Christian teachings that forbade killing, infanticide was replaced in Europe, to a great extent, by the practice of abandonment. Unwanted newborns were abandoned on the doorsteps of private homes, at crossroads, in marketplaces, or in the wilderness. Although abandonment did not involve direct killing, few abandoned newborns were found and raised (usually, though not always, as slaves), and most consequently died.

By the Middle Ages, Christianity had created another alternative to infanticide and abandonment: oblation, or turning over unwanted children to monasteries to be reared by and eventually to join the celibate religious orders. Because a dowry was frequently required, oblation was not always an option for those of modest means. Later, perhaps in response to increased demand, the Catholic Church established "foundling hospitals," which allowed women to abandon children to their care anonymously, by means of a turntable in the hospital wall and a bell that would alert the staff. First created in Italy, these institutions soon spread to other Christian countries in Europe.

When the Reformation began in the sixteenth century, Protestants—who had no celibate religious orders to raise abandoned children—placed the responsibility of the economic support of an unwanted child on the father and the responsibility for the child's daily care on the unwed mother, who would thus have a permanent public reminder of her sin. In Catholic regions, unwed mothers were forced to surrender their children to foundling hospitals, where child mortality was usually many times higher than in the general population. As punishment for their sin, they were also forced to breastfeed other people's children for one year. Foundling hospitals were later taken over by the various states, but as demand increased and child mortality decreased in the nineteenth century (creating an explosion in the number of unwanted children that the states were unable to support), they disappeared.

From this historical perspective, it is clear why concrete references to abortion are few in the first six centuries of Christianity and merely episodic (and certainly not a matter of heated debate) until the late nineteenth century. Until the twentieth century, when growing numbers of unwanted pregnancies and the introduction of safer methods made abortion increasingly popular, abortion was not a major public health problem. It is clear, however, that throughout history, Christian teachings embraced a predominantly negative view of abortion and contraception, which were, in fact, generally considered to be sins.

Christian Values about Abortion
(Gudorf, 2003; Dombrowski and Deltete, 2000)

Two Catholic philosophers, Daniel. A. Dombrowski and Robert Deltete (2000), reviewing the Catholic Church's opposition to abortion, conclude that throughout history it has been based on two arguments: the *perversity position* and the *ontological position.* The most traditional argument was the perversity position, which predominated almost un-contested until the seventeenth century. The perversity position starts from the premise that abortion is a perversion of the true and only func-tion of sex. Sexual intercourse was considered moral only if performed as a means for procreation within marriage. Abortion is a sin because it interferes with this purpose.

The restriction of the purpose of sexuality to procreation is attributed to the early influence of Stoicism, which taught that humans should con-trol their emotions with reason. Furthermore, the quest of religion, which accepted the Greco-Roman duality of matter and spirit, was to save the soul imprisoned in the body. Thus, "in the hierarchy of virtues, martyr-dom, virginity and celibacy led the way. Marriage that was committed to sexual abstinence was more holy than marriage in which spouses had intercourse for the sake of procreation. There was no good simply in the pleasure of sex," and "the value of fetal life did not need to be discussed; it was assumed as the God-given product of sexual activity, designed" only for that purpose (Albrecht, 2003, p. 87). This line of thought may explain why the religious penalties were frequently less severe for abortion than for contraception and less severe still for sterilization.

Applied today, this traditional perspective would condemn all forms of contraception, including the rhythm method (which is currently ac-cepted by the Catholic Church) and would also condemn postmeno-pausal intercourse as well as intercourse for anyone who is sterile. The traditional perversity position was officially rejected during the II Vatican Council, which met from 1962 to 1965, which agreed that marriage had two equally important primary purposes: procreation and the unity of the spouses. It was understood that the purpose of unity included the enjoyment of sex for nonprocreative purposes. After this solemn agreement (Vatican Councils have authority equal to that of the Pope), it was expected that the Catholic Church would fully accept contraception. After considerable internal debate, however, the papacy accepted only "natural methods" of contraception, based on periodic sexual abstinence during the woman's fertile period.

This decision seems compatible with a recent, milder version of the perversity position stating that sex is moral within marriage as long as it leaves open the possibility of pregnancy. Implicit in this position is that natural methods allow for the possibility that the woman will become pregnant if it is God's will, a very real possibility, given the relatively high failure rate of these methods. Unexplained is why the principle does not apply to modern contraceptives, which also have significant failure rates.

Based on the same principle was one of the teachings of the Medical School of the Catholic University in Chile. José Barzelatto recalls that when he was a medical student there, he was taught that it was morally acceptable to use a condom during intercourse to collect a semen sample for diagnostic purposes, provided that it was pinpricked before use. Masturbation, even for this purpose, was unacceptable.

In contrast to the perversity position, the key to the ontological position for opposing abortion is the status of the embryo/fetus during the pregnancy: At what stage of development are we dealing with an individual or a person? When does the new being merit full respect as a human being that has a soul and a body? How does its value compare with that of the pregnant woman? These are some of the questions that have concerned Christian theologians throughout history, and the answers have created controversies that persist to this day. During the first centuries of Christianity, the few texts that referred directly to abortion considered it a very serious sin, a form of murder. By the fifth century, theologians were making a distinction between abortion and homicide, both sins but with different penalties. This distinction was linked to whether or not the fetus was formed (ensouled). This way of thinking had been influenced by pre-Christian Aristotelian philosophy: You cannot be something unless you have the form and the attributes of that object or being, although you may have the potential to become it. The classic example is that of pieces of wood, which are not a table but which can be made into a table. Aristotle also believed that all living beings had a body and a soul, or principle of life.

Aristotle recognized the need for the interaction of a male component and a female component—semen and menstrual blood, in his words—to create an entity that would initiate the reproductive process. He compared this entity to a seed or an egg and proposed that if it was not lost, as he believed most were, but was retained for up to "seven days (within the woman) then it is certain that conception has taken place" (quoted in Ford, 1988, p. 27). This is remarkably parallel to what we now know about the formation of the zygote and implantation. Aristotle's limited knowledge of embryology, however, led him to the false belief that he could recognize a male fetus after forty days of gestation and a female fetus after ninety days.

Aristotle described three stages in the development of the embryo/fetus: Prior to forty days of gestation (for males) or ninety days of gestation (for females), there was an unformed being that, like a plant, had a *vegetative soul*. Once a formed fetus was visible, including recognizable external genitalia, a *sensitive soul* had taken over. Finally, at a time that Aristotle did not claim to know, a *rational soul* arrived from outside, making the human fetus capable of enjoying *vegetative, sensitive,* and *rational* life. Aristotle was adamant that abortions should be performed before sensation and human life began—that is, sometime before forty days for males or 90 days for females. Later we discuss the influence of Aristotle's thoughts on the teachings of Islam.

Aristotle's account remained virtually unchallenged for about two thousand years and acquired great weight in Christian Europe. In the thirteenth century, the influential theologian Saint Thomas Aquinas championed this way of thinking with an important difference. In his view, it was an act of God that created the human intellective soul within the fetus, which occurred at forty days for males and ninety days for females (Ford, 1988). Other theologians proposed later dates for human ensoulment, but in their contact with the faithful, priests referred to ensoulment at quickening, or when the woman first feels the fetus moving in her womb (about the beginning of the fifth month of pregnancy). Quickening is also called *fetal animation* (movement), a terms that derives from the Latin *anima*, or "soul."

This theory of late ensoulment, also known as *delayed hominization*, impacted the discussions of abortion by allowing less-severe penalties for early abortions and by raising questions about whether abortions before ensoulment should be morally permissible under certain circumstances. In fact, some early Christian texts justified abortion under specific circumstances, most frequently to save the woman's life and particularly, but not exclusively, in early pregnancy. A prominent fifteenth-century advocate of this view was Antoninus, an archbishop of Florence whom the Vatican not only refrained from criticizing but also later declared a saint (Maguire, 2001). Ecclesiastical penalties for abortion tended to increase with the duration of the pregnancy and were usually less severe than those indicated for homicide; however, a few reputable penitential books (lists of penances for sins) stipulated higher penalties for abortion and even contraception than for murder.

The opposing theory states that ensoulment occurs at the time of conception. In the seventeenth century, this theory, known as *immediate hominization,* was supported by a popular but mistaken scientific school of thought: the *preformation theory.* The preformation theory—which derived from the first glimpses of the microscopic world—proposed that all parts of the body already existed in (according to some scientists) the sperm or (according to other scientists) the egg, and the parts simply had to grow and become visible. Some scientists even imagined that, with the help of the microscope, they could see a little human being bundled inside the head of the spermatozoon.

The Catholic Church officially accepted the theory of delayed hominization until 1854, when Pope Pius IX proclaimed the dogma of the Immaculate Conception, implicitly endorsing the view that life started at conception. This position was further confirmed in 1869, when the Catholic Church formally eliminated any distinction between a formed and an unformed fetus by punishing all abortions with excommunication.

The Current Position of the Catholic Church

The sin of cooperating with an abortion now carries the maximum Catholic penalty: excommunication (deprivation of the rights of church membership, including access to the sacraments). The Code of Canon Law of 1917 explicitly stated that this penalty would be imposed on the woman who aborts as well as on those who perform the procedure (Callahan, 1970; Dombrowski and Deltete, 2000). In 1983 this penalty was reinforced by the promulgation of a new Catholic Code of Canon Law, which lists abortion and violent attack on the body of the Pope as the only two acts that incur automatic excommunication (Gudorf, 1998).

This position of the Catholic Church is based on its acceptance of the zygote, embryo, or fetus as a full human being, from the time of fertilization, and on the view that there is absolutely no moral justification for taking an innocent life. This position rejects the notion that during early pregnancy a "potential" human being exists and accepts instead the notion that from the "moment" of fertilization, there exists a "full" human being with human potential that will continue to develop in the womb and throughout his or her lifetime.

Automatic excommunication does not apply to the killing of another human being. Thus, the Catholic Church condemns abortion more severely than murder, including infanticide. Furthermore, excommunication does not apply to those who are under eighteen years of age or to persons who have no real alternative (that is to say, those who, in clear conscience, are absolutely convinced that they have no better option). A survey done in Colombia showed that 84 percent of priests did not excommunicate the women who confessed to having had an abortion (Munera, 1994). The implication of this study is that the priests made the judgment (normally reserved for a bishop) that most women who aborted were absolutely convinced that they had no better option. This finding matches our own experience: We have repeatedly heard from Latin American women that they know which priests in their area will hear them in confession and approve of their use of modern contraceptives, although officially forbidden by the Catholic Church.

The anti-abortion position is one of the Catholic Church's solemn teachings, but it is not a dogma. As far as the Catholic Church is concerned, when the Pope formally states that a teaching is a dogma, this view is infallible—that is to say, it can never change. In contrast, although a solemn teaching carries great weight, it is subject to the possibility of future change. In fact, for at least four decades, many Catholic moral theologians have argued in favor of expanding the circumstances that could make an abortion a moral decision. A frequently raised example is the presence of severe congenital fetal malformations that are incompatible with life, such as anencephalia (the absence of the upper portion of the central nervous system). Why not allow women to terminate a pregnancy that, if carried to term, will result in the delivery of a child who is able to survive no more than a few hours?

A different example of dissent is set forth in a book by a prominent Catholic theologian and published with the approval (imprimatur) of the Vatican. The author strictly opposes abortion but argues nevertheless that because of the possibility of twinning (see Chapter 2 herein), a new individual cannot begin until the primitive streak appears. In response to the question that is the title of his book—When did I begin?—his life could not have begun until two weeks after fertilization (Ford, 1988).

It is also pertinent to note that the Catholic Church does not currently require that fetuses be baptized; in fact, until 1895 it was forbidden to do so. Furthermore, according to Saint Augustine, the unborn would not rise on Resurrection Day (Maguire, 2001).

Interestingly, Catholics around the world seem to have as many abortions as do non-Catholics. In the United States, statistics show that Catholic women have abortions at the same rate as all other women in the population but at a higher rate than Protestant women (Jones, Darroch, and Henshaw, 2002). Furthermore, in countries with predominantly Catholic populations, such as the nations of Latin America, abortion rates are not lower (Requena, 1965). A survey carried out among 1,239 Catholic women in an abortion clinic in Colombia showed that 60 percent acknowledged that they were at risk of being excommunicated by the Catholic Church, but 65 percent did not consider abortion a grave mortal sin, and 82 percent believed that God would not forsake them for what they were doing. "He will understand my problem" was their standard answer (Munera, 1994).

The hierarchy of the Catholic Church clearly opposes the interruption of the reproductive process starting from fertilization, but this position is contested within the Catholic Church and disregarded by a large proportion of its followers. By its action, the Catholic laity is (consciously or subconsciously) exercising two traditional practices of the Catholic Church: *probabilism* and *respect for individual conscience.* The principle of probabilism states that "given theological doubt about the application of a moral law, one may follow any probable opinion of a theological expert" (Gudorf, 2003, p. 71). The principle of *respect for individual conscience* refers to a position that Catholic authorities have repeatedly affirmed: The voice of conscience must be obeyed even if it is not always a reliable guide to moral good.

Exceptions to the Rule—Direct and Indirect Action

The previously described position notwithstanding, the Catholic Church accepts abortion under two circumstances: when the pregnancy is ectopic and when it coexists with a cancer of the genital organs. Following a very old philosophical moral distinction between *direct* and *indirect* actions, the Catholic Church (as we have seen) severely condemns "direct" abortions, or the direct killing of the embryo or the fetus. Nevertheless, by applying the doctrine of double effect, the Catholic Church accepts inducing an "indirect" abortion to save the life of the woman (Beauchamp and Childress, 1994). This rule states, in summary, that if an action has a good and a bad effect (in this case saving the life of the woman but causing the death of the fetus), the act is not forbidden as long as there is no intention of doing harm, even when that harm is foreseeable. In practical terms, it means that if removing an organ is required to save the life of a woman, that act is acceptable even if there is an embryo or fetus inside that organ. Although the final result will be the death of the fetus, that was not the primary intention of the procedure. As far as the Catholic Church is concerned, there are only two situations in which this rule can be applied:

- A pregnant woman has cancer of the cervix, and a hysterectomy (surgical removal of the uterus), which will result in the death of the fetus, can save her life.
- A woman has an ectopic pregnancy (a live embryo implanted in the fallopian tube instead of in the uterus), which could lead to her death, but extirpation of the tube with the embryo inside can save her life.

In contrast, the Catholic Church does not accept the termination of a pregnancy to save a woman's life by directly removing only the embryo/fetus, as in the examples that follow:

- A pregnant woman suffers from severe cardiac disease, which could kill her if the pregnancy is not terminated.
- A pregnant woman has a premature rupture of membranes that leads to a severe uterine infection in the fifth month of gestation. The fetus is still alive, but the infection will spread and kill the woman in hours if the uterine contents are not removed.

With modern technology, a tubal ectopic pregnancy can be diagnosed before it ruptures the tube and can be surgically treated by opening the tube and extracting only the embryo, thus preserving not only the woman's life but also her future fertility. However, this would presumably be considered a direct abortion by the Catholic Church. Consequently, Catholics may interpret this to mean that they should wait until the tube ruptures and then proceed with an indirect abortion, even though this will put the woman's fertility, indeed her life, at great risk. This position is taken in some Catholic hospitals in Latin America, even though the embryo will always die.

It is difficult to find significant moral differences between direct and indirect abortions. In all cases, the act is an intervention intended to save the woman's life, which is considered of greater value than the life of the fetus. The argument that there is no justification because the end (to save the life of the woman) does not justify the means (the direct killing of the fetus) is certainly debatable, particularly when the fetus will inevitably be lost.

The difficulty of explaining the double-effect rule in a convincing way without weakening the argument that rejects abortion as an absolute principle may explain why in public debates Catholic pro-life advocates avoid the subject of the Catholic Church's moral acceptance of indirect abortion.

Protestant Perspectives on Abortion (Albrecht, 2003)

Protestantism, a sect of Christians who are neither under the authority of the Roman Catholic Church nor part of the Eastern Orthodox Christian churches, comprises such a diverse variety of denominations that it is difficult to summarize the values they bring to bear on abortion. Moreover, when the Reformation began in the sixteenth century, abortion does not appear to have been an issue of major concern. Neither Luther nor Calvin more than mentions abortion. In Geneva, where Calvin exerted great influence over the laws of the city, the civil laws of the time did not refer to abortion. Luther's statement that the law should allow the conscience to act freely, which was actually made with reference to legislation on marriage and divorce rather than with reference to abortion, was one of his important contributions (Pérez Aguirre, 2000).

At present, good and bad are not as absolute for Protestants as they are for Catholics. Traditionally, the emphasis has been on individuals to look into their faith and assume responsibility for their relationship with God. In general, Protestants accepted the sexual ethics that they inherited from Catholicism; including the idea that procreation was the purpose of sexuality. On one hand, though, Protestants took a more conservative stance toward abortion than the Catholic Church's acceptance of late hominization, by arguing for the full humanity of the fetus from its earliest stage. On the other hand, they took a more liberal position than the Roman Catholics by regarding marriage as a normal state for all adults, including their ministers.

During the following centuries, Protestantism evolved with respect to its views on sexuality and procreation. Appreciation of sex within marriage for purposes of companionship as well as reproduction were typical for groups such as the Puritans in the early seventeenth century, but it was not until the nineteenth century that the practice of contraception began to increase and birth rates began to decrease among Protestants. Even among the devout, many did not consider withdrawal as illicit and periodic abstinence had always been practiced for birth control. In addition, condoms and potions that claimed to induce abortion were used among the less devout. As Western societies became increasingly industrialized and urban and as child mortality decreased, the concept of the family changed, and contraception became widely practiced and accepted by most Protestants. In the twentieth century, Protestant ministers—as husbands and fathers, as well as pastors—joined others in first obtaining the acceptance of contraception within their churches and later reversing the laws against contraception. Support for the legalization of abortion came more slowly. "By the 1970s in the U.S. major mainline Protestant denominations would endorse, not abortion per se, but the need for women to be able to exercise the freedom of their own consciences in the difficult decisions necessitated by unwanted pregnancies." Included was support for the use of public funds to ensure "full and equal access to contraception and abortion to all women, regardless of race, age and economic standing" (Albrecht, 2003, p. 94, 95).

In general, because Protestants agreed on the sacredness of fetal life, they had serious reservations about pregnancy termination. They did not, however, give the same value to the life of the fetus as to the life of the woman. In other words, in the Protestant view, a human life is developing from the very beginning of pregnancy that merits great respect, but not on a basis equivalent to the respect or rights due to a fully developed person.

As evident in the statement made by the Lutheran Women's Caucus, Protestants also relate their analysis of abortion to issues of social justice: "The incidence of abortion could be greatly reduced with social and cultural changes for which we all have responsibility, including complete and accurate sex education, adequate and available contraception, responsible non-coercive sexuality, health care, child care, parental leave, and other social support." It also called upon their "various church bodies to work actively for the social and cultural changes that will reduce the incidence of abortion and stop scapegoating women who have abortions" (Albrecht, 2003, p. 96).

Nevertheless, some Protestants, mostly Evangelicals, have played leadership roles in the staunchly conservative U.S. Christian Coalition, which has been increasingly visible in the national political arena in its promotion of changes in legislation and government regulations designed to restrict or eliminate access to abortion.

Jewish Perspectives on Abortion (Zoloth, 2003)

Jewish religious norms are based on a reasoned analysis of the religion's sacred texts as applied to changing circumstances. As Laurie Zoloth puts it, "When new historical situations arise, and the daily enactment of community and faithfulness shifts against political, scientific, or physical contingencies, a process of heightened discourse reshapes the new enactments." "For Jews, the cultural and economic realities of modernity affect religious practice, social justice, and ethical norms. Family life, families, childrearing, and sexuality are part of the practice of religion" (2003, p. 22).

The debates that result from this continuous discussion, whose intention is to adapt the commandments to changing circumstances, have been recorded throughout time and serve as guidance for new discussions. The Talmud codified the debates that took place over the course of seven hundred years, starting at about 200 B.C. Jewish law has developed during the centuries since, based on the responses (*responsa*) of religious scholars to new questions about the Talmud posed throughout the years. The result is an abundant literature that records centuries of disagreement rather than consensus.

Abortion appears as an option for Jewish women from the earliest sources of both the Bible and the Talmud. According to Jewish thought, abortion is morally justified under certain circumstances, such as when the woman's life or her physical or mental health is at risk. In such cases, abortion becomes a moral obligation, giving the higher priority to the life and health of the woman than to the fetus. The moral status of the fetus, according to Jewish tradition, progresses with gestational age and proximity to viability, but the fetus is not considered to become a full person until birth (traditionally when the head of the newborn emerges from the birth canal).

With respect to abortion, the discussion and commentary take one of two courses: Either (1) the fetus is part of the body of a woman and does not, therefore, have an equal moral claim, or (2) according to a later understanding put forward by Maimonides in the twelfth century, in cases where a pregnancy is endangering the life or health of a woman, the fetus can be considered a *rodef* (an aggressor, literally one who pursues), which may be killed as a permitted act of self-defense. The decision is to be made by the woman in conjunction with a rabbi, as her spiritual teacher.

At present, "among Orthodox Jews, only saving the life of the woman can justify abortion. Among Conservative and Reform Jews, the health and welfare of the woman are also relevant and maternal welfare can include various social and psychological considerations. Because for Jews the fetus is understood as on the path to becoming a person, it is never of negligible worth, and abortion requires moral justification" (Gudorf, 1998, p. 2).

Muslim Perspectives on Abortion (Shaikh, 2003)

The Koran, the collected revelations of Allah to Muhammad and the fundamental authority for Muslims, is very explicit in describing a progressive development of the fetus in three stages that are very similar to those described by Aristotle. The fetus is considered a whole human being when it is "ensouled"—that is, when the angel breathes the spirit into it, most frequently considered to take place at 120 days of pregnancy. The Koran does not discuss abortion explicitly but condemns the killing of one's own children. Infanticide (as we have seen) was the main concern in Muhammad's time. The Koran also establishes that "damages paid to the father of a fetus expelled in an accident before the fifth month are only 1/10th of those for a person, but after the fifth month, full damages are due" (Gudorf, 1998, p. 2). These Koranic teachings explain why almost all Muslim schools of thought forbid abortion in general after 120 days but accept it at any time if the pregnant woman's life is in danger. In the interpretation of some scholars, late abortions are also justified in the presence of a severely malformed fetus.

In relation to abortion prior to ensoulment, there are four classic Islamic positions:

1. Unconditional permission to terminate a pregnancy without justification, up to 120 days of gestational age: This view is adopted by the Zaydi school and by some Hanafi and Shafi'i scholars. The Hanbali school allows abortion through the use of oral drugs within 40 days of conception.

2. Up to 120 days, conditional permission to abort when there is acceptable justification: Abortion without a valid reason is disapproved (*makruh*) but not forbidden (*haram*). This is the opinion of the majority of Hanafi and Shafi'i scholars.

3. Abortion is always strongly disapproved (*makruh*). This is the view held by some Maliki jurists.

4. Abortion is unconditionally prohibited (*haram*). This reflects the other Maliki view, as well as the Zahiri, Ibadiyya, and Imamiyya schools of legal thought. These Zahiri, Ibadiyya, and Imamiyya schools have a limited following within Islam.

This diversity, which contrasts with the wide acceptance of contraception, suggests a flexibility in the way that Muslim societies have historically approached the issue of abortion. The extensive discussions about abortion-inducing potions in the medical manuals of classical Islam also suggest that abortion was a part of social reality in ancient times. Islam, which teaches the sanctity of human life, shows a profound respect for the potential for human life, but the concern for the fetus is considered within the larger context of the woman, the family, and the society.

This view explains some recent events: In Egypt the Grand Sheikh of Al-Azhar, Sayed Tantawi, supported a *fatwa* allowing abortion in cases of rape and affirmed the woman's right to privacy. In Iran, two *fatwas* were issued: one by the Ayatollah Ali Khameni in favor of abortion for fetuses under 10 weeks if they tested positive for thalassemia (a genetic blood disorder) and another by the Grand Ayatolla Yusuf Saanei in favor of abortion in the first trimester for reasons that included the woman's health and fetal abnormalities. In the same spirit, in a 1995 submission to the South African parliament, the Judicial Committee of the Islamic Council of South Africa recognized the right to terminate a pregnancy before 120 days for reasonable cause, including the impairment of the mental capacity or the integrity of the woman and the inability or unwillingness of the woman to accept the responsibility of parenthood. Given the historical diversity, it is not surprising that other contemporary Muslim societies have shown a tendency to adopt a more rigid approach.

Hindu Perspectives on Abortion (Jain, 2003)

India's ancient religion, Hinduism, is properly known as the San-natan Dharma, or the Eternal Tradition. The most important sacred texts are the Vedas, which are accepted by scholars to have preceded the Christian Era by many centuries. Hinduism, which has been seen as more of a confederation of religions than a dogmatically unified system, is characterized by rejection of absolutism and by understanding that the universe is in a continuous process of change. Thus, although *Dharma* is seen as the cosmic law, it is not static; it is characterized by movement, dynamism, and the capacity to adapt to changing situations. *Dharma* is often compared to a river, which has permanence and continuity but is never the same. This continuous change is seen as the immutable cosmic law, which must be accepted and experienced without fear. The balance between universal values and consideration of individual circumstances is essential to Hinduism. Applied to moral dilemmas, this balance trans-lates into acceptance and encouragement for individuals that must be guided by the needs and challenges of each particular case.

The concept that the soul is eternal and indestructible is another fundamental principle of Hindu thought. After death, the soul moves from one life to the next in a continuity of rebirth and transmigration. Human life—the highest form of life, attained after innumerable cycles of birth and rebirth—gives the human being the opportunity to realize the self and merge with the *Atman* (godhead). The accumulated effects of good and bad actions during the numerous lives are called *karma,* which the soul carries from one life to the next. Each life is an opportunity to improve one's karma; death can provide the possibility of rebirth closer to the godhead. To reach *moksha*—to be freed from the continuous process of births and deaths by merging the self to the Atman—is the supreme achievement (Jain, 2003). "Moksha requires living through a number of lives since one can only achieve moksha from the status of a male Brahmin. (Brahmins are the highest caste of the Hindu caste system)" (Gudorf, 1998, p. 1).

Although the status of women has varied throughout the Hindu tra-dition, the purpose of marriage has remained to maintain the continuity of the family. Because the soul is incorporated in the new living entity from the very beginning of embryonic life, Hinduism ideally rejects abortion, which will abruptly interrupt the natural process of transmi-gration from one being to another before it has the chance to improve its karma.

Hinduism's traditional rejection of absolutism makes it intrinsically well equipped to address a scale of competing rights and values. Thus, in pregnancies where the woman risks grave injury or even death, perhaps because the adult human being is karmically more evolved than the human embryo or fetus, the *Charak Samhita* accords greater weight to the life of the woman than to the life of the fetus. The preference of the life and health of the woman is illustrated in the *Susruta Samhita* (a treatise devoted primarily to surgery), which "recommends abortion . . . [when] the fetus is defective, and the chances of a normal delivery are negligible." Susruta suggests that in these instances, "the surgeon should not wait for nature to take its course but should intervene by performing craniotomy operations to remove the fetus" (Jain, 2003, p. 136); that is to say, it recommends what some now call a partial-birth abortion.

The concepts described are reflected in the 1971 Indian MTP Act, which permits abortion in cases of rape, incest, and even threats to the mental health of the woman (which may include the birth of an unwanted child). Given these broad terms, abortion is available virtually on demand. The government of India is planning to liberalize the law even further, by extending abortion rights to those under eighteen years of age, without the consent of their guardians, in order to prevent adolescents from resorting to the unsafe abortions that claim numerous lives every year. The draft legislation circulated to state governments has elicited no Hindu religious opposition.

Buddhist Perspectives on Abortion (Suwanbubba, 2003)

Because Buddhism began as an offshoot of Hinduism, many of the philosophical underpinnings of Hinduism also apply to Buddhism. Buddhism, however, sought reform by rejecting the authority of the various existing Hindu religions. Like Hinduism, Buddhism is not organized around a central authority and Buddhist teaching may vary from one country to another.

Buddhism, like Hinduism, accepts that karma is transferred from one life to the next but rejects the concept that anything is permanent, including the self. "The goal of Buddhism is to attain liberation (nirvana) from the unhappiness and pain inherent in worldly existence . . . caused by uncontrollable desires for pleasure and satisfaction. . . . The way to liberation is by accepting that everything is ephemeral," so that "self-centered desire can be abandoned"; by cultivating "a detached attitude" and rejecting violence, "unhappiness can be eliminated. . . . The final goal is not a paradise or a heavenly world. Nirvana is an everlasting state of happiness and peace to be reached here on earth" (Sachedina, 1989, pp. 2, Buddhism chapter).

"The essential Buddhist teaching is that we suffer and cause others to suffer because of greed, ill-will and delusion," the "three roots of evil," also known as the three poisons (Loy, 2002, p. 249). In order to be happy, one must transform these into generosity, compassion, and wisdom. Buddhism gives less weight to the concept of evil than to its causes. Whereas Abrahamic religions (Judaism, Christianity, and Islam) tend to emphasize the struggle between good and evil, Buddhism emphasizes the opposition between ignorance and enlightenment. For Abrahamic religions, to be on the side of good or evil depends on our will, and the basic issue is which side we are on. In contrast, Buddhism understands that the basic issue is our self-knowledge, our understanding of what really motivates us (Loy, 2002).

Buddhism's emphasis on detachment and nonviolence impacts attitudes toward reproduction and sexuality. In Buddhism, marriage is not a religious ritual; in fact, it is seen as inferior to the pursuance of monastic life. Marriage and sexuality are seen as positive as long as sexual misconduct is not involved (such as being unfaithful to one's partner, having sex with someone who has been ordained, or having sex with a women who is under the protection of her parents).

Although Buddhist scriptures are silent on the subject of abortion, in the context of their philosophy and given the emphasis on nonviolence and the continuity of life, we can assume disapproval of abortion. "Buddhism views the formation of life as having a real continuity since the karmic force directly links the moment of death with the moment of new appearance (rebirth)" (Sachedina, 1989, p. 5, Buddhism chapter). The thread is continuous, so there is no time or space before the embryo becomes human and the object of respect. Nevertheless, Buddhism stresses that universal norms (*dharmas*) should not conflict with human nature. The doctrine of the Middle Path asserts that although the universal norms of human life are constant, the ways of applying them vary. General principles must be adapted to the infinitely varying circumstances of actual life. Middle Path is described as not too much, not too little, not too tight, not too loose. That is to say, moderation in all activities and in every aspect of life, without extreme austerity or extreme indulgence, is recommended. (Suwanbubba, 2003). An "abortion law that allows, but does not compel, abortion when the life or health of the woman is in danger or for reason of rape, enables the woman and her physician to follow the 'Middle Path'" (Sachedina, 1989, p. 9, Buddhism chapter).

In Thai Buddhism, intention is key. In cases of abortions with good intentions, the terms of retribution or negative karma effects would be less, but even among abortions performed with good intentions, the negative effects will vary. For example, a late abortion would have more negative significance than an early one, and an abortion for sex selection (a bad intention) would have very serious negative effects (Suwanbubba, 2003).

In addition, it is important to take into account that in Buddhism the goal of religion and of the activities of monks is not to manipulate society by, for example, influencing government actions, but to improve their own spiritual status and that of others. This helps explain why the very liberal abortion laws of most Buddhist countries have not received significant political opposition from the Buddhist religious authorities. In the case of Japan, moreover, the traditional Japanese Shinto belief that the fetus does not have a spirit until coming into the light at birth encouraged the view that abortion was no more than a movement from darkness to darkness (Gudorf, 1998).

Chinese Perspectives on Abortion (Shang, 2003)

Throughout time, the three main Chinese religions, Confucionism, Taoism, and (later) Chinese Buddhism, have all contributed to the development of the Chinese concept of universal harmony. This is not only a religious belief but also a philosophical and sociopolitical ideal within which family values are greatly celebrated. For thousands of years, the Chinese have believed that reproduction, sexuality, and family life could gravely affect the balance, order, and harmony of human society and the natural world. This traditional belief in universal harmony is instrumental to an understanding of the general acceptance of recent government policies, including the rapid adoption of modern contraceptive practices and abortion, that are designed to control population growth.

Although abortion was not encouraged in Chinese tradition, there was no explicit code forbidding it, and it has been employed under various circumstances since ancient times. A woman usually resorted to abortion when she was faced with a pregnancy considered disastrous or disgraceful—for instance, when the pregnancy was the result of prostitution, an affair, incest, or rape or when it put the woman's life in peril. Because abortion was considered unnatural and shameful, it was kept secret, but there was no significant religious condemnation, and—unless the act was seen as unnecessary—most people reacted with tolerance and compassion.

The "Table of Merits and Errors" from the Yuan Dynasty (1279–1368 C.E.) illustrates how abortion ranked as a misdeed in traditional China. Abortion is counted as a three-hundred-point error, the same as for enticing a person to gamble, whereas murder is ranked as a one-thousand-point error, and setting someone's house on fire is a five-hundred-point error. Infanticide (more accurately, female infanticide), practiced among low-income families of China from time immemorial, is listed as a one-thousand-point error. Clearly, the fetus was not considered to have the same value as an infant, child, or adult.

Moreover, Chinese religions have always given family and social values priority over the concerns of the individual. If abortion profits the family or society, then it is a reasonable act. If an adult must be ready to sacrifice his or her life for the family and society, why not a fetus? It is also worthwhile to note that the patriarchal Chinese family considered children to be part of the father's private property, and for most Chinese, a necessary abortion is a shameful but understandable matter of parental choice.

Is a Religious Consensus Possible?

This short review of the perspectives and values of some of the main religions of the world shows that, in general, religions have serious concerns about abortion. Although there are considerable differences in their teachings, there are also many similarities; the main similarity is that most of the religions allow abortion, under different circumstances and for different reasons, as a moral choice. Because, as we have seen, religious views about abortion have changed throughout history, it is reasonable to assume that they will continue to do so. The increasing global preference for small families, reflected in the dramatic drop in birth rates around the world, is changing sexual and reproductive behavior everywhere. Religions will have to continue to adapt to social changes as they have done throughout history.

Moreover, a shrinking world is bringing together people from different countries and from very different cultures. The expansion of and improvements in communications have allowed people who were distant and isolated to see and hear each other on their television sets. Increased travel and migration are bringing together persons of very different backgrounds. As a result, people must now find a rational way to explain their differences—including their religious values—to themselves and to others. Organized religions and theologians must also take part in this dialogue. The Genval consensus, which took place before the UN's Fourth International Conference on Population and Development (ICPD) in 1994, illustrates this increasing openness to dialogue and to the need for religious collaboration to improve social justice in a globalized world:

The Genval Consensus

Several people involved in the preparation of the ICPD anticipated a heated controversy on women's reproductive rights, particularly on the subject of abortion. Because the main opposition to women's reproductive freedom came from some religious groups, the importance of a prior discussion among theologians from different faiths about the agenda of the 1994 Cairo Conference on Population and Development became clear. Convened by the Park Ridge Center for the Study of Health, Faith and Ethics (Chicago) in collaboration with the International Forum for Biophilosophy (Louvain, Belgium), thirty-four theologians and scholars met as individuals, rather than as official representatives of their religions, in Genval, Belgium, in May 1994 (Park Ridge Center, 1994). In the selection of the invitees, personal prominence, diversity of position, and gender and geographical distribution were taken into consideration. Only eight women participated, but their presence served to highlight new interpretations about the role of women in their traditions and offered some of the male theologians their first opportunity to be questioned by women peers about interpretations of their own faith.

As the Genval report explains, the "gathering in Belgium was not intended to make a contribution to the theory of inter-religious dialogue. Instead, the intent was practical: to articulate the interests and witnesses of religious communities on the themes of the ICPD and to seek points of convergence on these urgent issues" (Park Ridge Center, 1994, p. 2). In this spirit, the participants arrived at a remarkable consensus on each of the points of the ICPD agenda. They started by recognizing the importance that all religions enjoy the freedom to propagate and practice their faith and, as a corollary, that all people enjoy the freedom not to be obliged to follow a religion or to be bound by it. They recognized that international bodies could not achieve anything of importance for the larger world community if they were not allowed to challenge the religious outlook of one or more faiths. In addition, they called for prudence on the part of all religious communities in that they should be free to guide their followers and to try to persuade nonfollowers but should also be ready to receive criticism when their practices offend others. The Genval report states, "The voice of any single faith should not carry so much weight as to stifle debate or paralyze action on the international agenda" (Park Ridge Center, 1994, p. 5).

With respect to women, they noted, "Many ancient religious texts and modern interpretations reflect cultures of male dominance and are construed as divine authorization for the subjugation of women." They also noted an increasing self-criticism on this matter among different traditions, making it likely that "the claims for the full human dignity of women in the private and public as well as sacred and secular spheres of life, therefore, will likely find increasing support among and within religious communities, even when the official position of a religious tradition is at variance with the views of the larger body. . . . The fundamental and universal rights of women as human beings can be expected to receive support from a broadening spectrum of religious communities." They agreed, "Women individually are also understood to have the freedom to exercise conscience in matters that have an impact on their survival, health, well-being and destiny. For this freedom to be meaningful, women need access to education, the resources for reproductive health, and opportunities for personal development and socioeconomic advancement" (Park Ridge Center, 1994, pp. 9, 10).

Their agreement with respect to abortion reads as follows:

> While abortion is universally treated as a serious moral and religious concern, it is treated differently among and within religious communities. Most religious traditions do not forbid abortion altogether, yet some limit the conditions under which it may be permitted. Others understand it as a matter that is to be left to the discretion of the individual in conformity with the dictates of personal conscience.
>
> The rationales for taking one position or another on abortion among and within religious groups include a commitment to the sanctity of human life even in its earliest embryonic stages; an interest in the current and future health and well-being of both the mother and the embryo or fetus; a respect for the right of a woman to act as a full moral agent; and a concern that the state not interfere in personal matters of conscience. Although some traditions and people of faith ground their stance in one of these rationales to the exclusion of the rest, many others develop positions that draw on several of these perspectives, resulting in a great

variety of assessments concerning when and under which circumstances abortion is morally justified.

Whatever their stance on abortion, religious communities cannot disregard the fact that it occurs and that, in places where abortion is illegal or heavily restricted, it often poses risk to the life and health of the woman. Decriminalization of abortion, therefore, is a minimal response to this reality and a reasonable means of protecting the life and health of women at risk.

Given the moral concern about abortion and the range of stances toward it taken by religious communities, the view of any particular religious tradition should not be imposed on others." (Park Ridge Center, 1994, pp. 14, 15)

The Genval consensus is a clear demonstration not only that a respectful dialogue among religions, maintaining intellectual integrity, is possible but also that agreement, even concerning matters as controversial as abortion, is possible. This opens wide the door for collaboration on the subject of abortion that will result in the reduction of pain and suffering for women.

The Chiang Mai Declaration

A more recent event expanded the possibility of such dialogue and collaboration among religions, by including women's organizations in a similar global effort. Between February 29 and March 3, 2004, forty-one religious and women's leaders participated in a "conversation" in Chiang Mai, Thailand, to discuss how, in an era of globalization, religions can play a more active role in advancing women's lives. The "conversation," was organized by the Center for Health and Social Policy and the Peace Council. The forty-one participants, who came from Africa, Asia, Latin America, the Middle East, Europe, and North America, unanimously adopted a far-ranging declaration that states in part:

- "We, the participants in this conference on women and religion, recognize that contemporary realities have tragic consequences for women's lives. Without a commitment to women's human rights and to the resolution of these tragedies, religions are failing the world. Their own relevance is at stake as they become more and more isolated from the values and needs of their members.

- It is urgent that religions address these realities." "Religions must no longer tolerate violence against women. Women are alienated from religions that do."
- "Religions at their best celebrate the dignity of each human being and of all life as valuable parts of a sacred whole. They inspire and empower us to compassion and justice. Religions, however, have not always been at their best. They have collaborated with dehumanizing values of cultural, economic, and political powers. Thus they have contributed to the suffering of women."
- "Religions can and must do better. They must reclaim their core values of justice, dignity, and compassion, and apply these values to women." (The Center for Health and Social Policy, 2004, pp. 9–11)

Specifically with respect to abortion, their unanimous declaration supported the Genval consensus by stating, "This is nowhere more evident than in the area of women's sexuality and reproductive health. Given the moral concern about abortion and the range of stances toward it, the view of any particular religious tradition should not be imposed on the consciences of others. Decriminalization of abortion is a minimal response to this reality" (The Center for Health and Social Policy, 2004, p. 12).

The Chiang Mai declaration concludes by saying that sharing "the same commitments to human dignity, social justice and human rights for all," the participants commit themselves "and call on other women and religious leaders to reach out to each other to enhance mutual understanding, support and cooperation" in order to "expand the consensus achieved" and "to define concrete, joint activities toward advancing women's human rights and well-being" in the belief "that when women and religious traditions collaborate, a powerful force for advancing women's human rights and leadership will be created" (Center for Health and Social Policy, 2004, p. 12).

The Teachings of Two Prominent Religious Leaders

We end this chapter by quoting two prominent religious leaders of our time, the Dalai Lama and Pope John Paul II.

The Dalai Lama has stated that "in the history of humanity there have been very tragic events which came about because of religion. Even to this day, we see that conflicts arise in the name of religion and the human community is further divided. If we were to meet this challenge, then I am sure we would find that there are enough grounds on which we can build harmony between the various religions and develop a genuine respect toward each other." He goes on to say, "After all, in humanity there are so many different mental dispositions, that simply one religion, no matter how profound, cannot satisfy all the variety of people." Acknowledging that most people recognize some religious background but that few live their lives as true believers, he concludes that "a variety of religions is actually necessary and useful and, therefore, the only sensible thing is that all different religions work together and live harmoniously, helping one another" (His Holiness the XIV Dalai Lama, 2001).

In his January 1, 1991, address "If You Want Peace, Respect the Conscience of Every Person," Pope John Paul II counseled respect for the "inalienable rights to follow one's own conscience and to profess and practice one's own faith. . . . People must not attempt to impose their own 'truth' on others. When religious law becomes synonymous with civil law, it can stifle religious freedom, even going so far as to restrict or deny other inalienable human rights. . . . Intolerance can also result from the recurring temptation to fundamentalism, which easily leads to serious abuses, such as the radical suppression of all public manifestations of diversity" (quoted in Sass, 1994).

These statements support our belief that the Genval report and the Chiang Mai declaration are in the mainstream of current religious thought and that a dialogue among religions that will identify common purposes is possible.

9
Ethical Values

Our Understanding of Ethics

You live in a country where a cruel dictatorship has taken over the national government. People "disappear" forever, or their corpses are found with clear signs of having been torturde to death. One night a dear friend knocks at your door saying that he cannot go back home because a police car is waiting for him in front of his house. You know that your friend is a student leader who has publicly expressed his opposition to the current government but has never been involved in any violent activity, much less any act that could be qualified as terrorism. You know him very well, and you can testify to his complete honesty. You receive him and offer refuge for as long as he wishes.

A few hours later the police come and ask if you know of this friend's whereabouts. Your ten-year-old son is there. You have taught him that he should never lie, even if telling the truth is painful. Truthfulness is a moral value to which you have always given first priority. You have to decide between (1) telling the truth and giving your friend up to face torture and possible death and (2) renouncing this principle on this particular occasion to follow your sense of justice and protect the life of a friend who is totally innocent of any wrongdoing.

This is an example of a personal moral problem or ethical dilemma, where the decision requires the person to weigh conflicting values in the light of specific circumstances and make a judgment about how to proceed. *Morals* and *ethics* are usually used as synonyms, and both refer to what is right and what is wrong, what is good and what is bad. Such personal decisions are in the realm of what we call our conscience or our personal values. In our everyday life, virtually every action we take involves a moral judgment; often it is made automatically, almost without reflection, but sometimes—as in actions related to abortion—it requires a quiet and prolonged analysis of all the values involved. Personal values should be weighed differently when the action affects only a few persons, such as when an abortion is requested or procured, than when the action affects society in general, such as when legislation about abortion is being considered.

Our personal values are the result of some instinctive knowledge of what is right or wrong, developed by our experiences throughout life and regulated by our social environment. Obviously, personal decisions should take into account not only personal benefits and consequences but also benefits and consequences for others and should be acted upon with total freedom. Other people's judgments of our actions may also be considered, but judgments that one person makes about the moral value of somebody else's actions are more, detached. They are usually guided by a general attitude toward a type of moral problem rather than by a judgment that considers the characteristics of a particular case and all the circumstances involved.

In order to protect the common good, societies must put some limits on the liberty of individuals to act according to their personal values. To set such limits, society must establish rules of conduct that are based on some agreed-upon guiding ethical principles. These agreed-upon principles are based on discussions of morality in the abstract that have, since antiquity, been a part of philosophy called ethics, which has attempted to develop guidelines and rules of moral behavior useful to both societies and individuals. Not surprisingly, a proliferation of ethical theories, sometimes contradictory but more commonly complementary, has developed throughout history.

Caution should be used when applying ethical principles because they do not provide fixed formulae for moral behavior applicable to individual circumstances but rather serve as the basis for individual and collective moral judgment. In many specific cases, ethical principles conflict with one another, and their application requires individual judgment. Moreover, one must also be aware that views about what is acceptable moral behavior have changed throughout history and vary from one society to another, influenced by different ethical theories and by changing circumstances. The debate continues on whether or not there are some universal ethical principles for all cultures, at any given time in history. We believe, as Ruth Macklin does, that certain basic ethical principles are universally accepted, although their application may vary from one society to another (Macklin, 1999).

The dynamism of the debate is stimulated by scientific progress. A clear example is found in the technological advances in the field of human reproduction, which have created new moral problems and the corresponding debate about how to apply ethical principles to them. Since the 1970s, this concern has resulted in the creation of the field of bioethics.

Ethicists and health professionals have developed a new ethical theory based on four principles that applies ethics to the field of health. Bioethics has enjoyed remarkable worldwide acceptance with respect to the professional conduct of health workers and discussions of health policies. A recent study by a distinguished Muslim scholar (Serour, 1994) found the four principles of bioethics compatible with the ethical teachings of the Sharia, the ancient Muslim law written in a different age and a different culture. Here we describe these four principles—*respect for persons, nonmaleficence, beneficence,* and *justice*—and discuss how we believe they apply to abortion. Because a lack of understanding of ethics has jeopardized access to abortion in some countries, including the United States, the discussion of ethics related to abortion is becoming increasingly relevant (Lazarus, 1997).

The Four Principles of Bioethics

1. The principle of *respect for persons* is also known as the principle of *autonomy*. Throughout this book we use the term *respect for person*s preferentially but not exclusively. This principle requires that each individual be acknowledged and treated as a free agent—this is to say that it be recognized that all individuals have full capacity for independent judgment and action when they face moral dilemmas. This principle recognizes *responsibility* as the central value of the moral act, which implies *knowledge* and *freedom* of action. The concept of *freedom* can be restricted only when it may harm someone else. *Respect for persons* mandates also the protection of individuals who are not fully autonomous, such as children, the mentally handicapped, and prisoners. The most common practical medical expression of the principle of *respect*

for persons is *informed consent. This is a process that* ensures that physicians fully inform their patients of alternative treatment possibilities and allow their patients the *freedom* to make the final decision based on full *knowledge* of the expected effect of the actions to be taken.

2. The principle of *nonmaleficence* correlates to the traditional medical rule of "do no harm." This obligation is far from being an absolute in medicine, where relative risk is a frequent consideration, meaning that there is a level of harm that can be tolerated to achieve the good pursued. A simple example that illustrates this kind of conflict is observed when a physician is confronted with the need to amputate a leg that has a malignant tumor in order to save the person's life.

3. The principle of *beneficence* builds on the previous principle, establishing the obligation to do good and to balance benefits against risks and costs. In other words, it is not enough to prevent or eliminate the bad; it is also necessary to promote the good. Maximize benefits and minimize harm is the basic principle of *utilitarianism,* a school of ethical thought that accepts as ethically correct those actions and social policies that produce the greatest benefit for the largest number of people.

    Respect for persons and the obligation to do good can be at odds with each other. A woman with severe hypertension late in pregnancy may need immediate delivery by cesarean section to preserve her life (*obligation to do good*), but she may refuse to undergo delivery by cesarean section (*respect for persons*). There is no easy solution to this kind of conflict as each of the individuals involved should act according to his/her conscience, depending on the particular circumstances of each case. Situations of conflict, as in the example given, require special attention from physicians so that they do not fall into ethically unacceptable paternalistic roles. Paternalistic actions deliberately go against a person's wishes in the guise of looking out for his or her own good or avoiding harm. An example of improper paternalistic behavior occurred several years ago in certain maternity hospitals in a Latin American country, where immediately after delivery an IUD was inserted in more than 90 percent of the women for the purpose of ensuring an appropriate interval between pregnancies (*intention to do good*). It is highly unlikely that over 90% of these women really wanted to use an IUD as a contraceptive or even wanted to use contraception at all (failure to have *respect for persons*).

4. The ethical principle of *justice* is a social concept based on *equity* and centered on the fair distribution of cost and benefits without distinction of gender, race, age, or socioeconomic status. *Justice* should be respected as the right of all individuals and as society's obligation toward them. This being the case, the application of the principle of *justice* requires *solidarity*. It should be understood that voluntary donations made by one or more individuals in the form of charity are not a substitute for the collective obligation of ensuring *justice*. Therefore, a *just* society requires the *solidarity* of its members.

    Another possible source of confusion is considering *equity* as synonymous with *equality*. Distributive *equity* proposes that each person has the right to a minimum of goods and services, commensurate with the available collective resources. This is different from a proposal that all material goods be distributed in equal portions to each person.

Given the broad generality of these four ethical principles, their application may vary among cultures that give different weight to each (Macklin, 1999). Because, as we have seen in the examples, the principles frequently conflict with one another when applied to a concrete situation, cultural variations should come as no surprise. When principles conflict, it must always be remembered that all four have their limits, while at the same time they are complementary. Furthermore, taking into account the socio-cultural context and the unique characteristics of each particular situation can enrich the criteria used to apply the principles. This includes a solid knowledge of the situation in question, of the facts and circumstances, and of the motivations of the players.

Because there is no agreed-upon hierarchical order for the ethical principles and the particular circumstances of an individual case can influence the priority given to each, it is difficult to resolve conflicts among them. The idea that one ethical principle should always override another is therefore unacceptable. Moreover, while there is general agreement on the need to accept well-justified exceptions to the application of any of these ethical principles, the interpretation of what constitutes a "well-justified exception" may vary widely.

The different weights given to these principles and the potential for internal conflicts among them explain why ethical principles are most valuable as *instruments for analysis* and *guides for action* rather than as prescriptive rules for individual decisions in moral problem solving.

The Bioethical Principles Applied to Abortion

Ethical reflection and bioethical principles help people to act with the greatest possible moral integrity. As we have seen, this may refer to a specific personal situation, such as seeking or providing an abortion, or to decisions that affect society as a whole, such as legislating on abortion. At an individual level, as in the physician-patient relationship, it is predominantly the first three principles that come into play: *respect for persons, nonmaleficence,* and *beneficence.* The situation for legislators is very different, because they must decide when people in their society should be penalized for individual actions. Their focus is on protecting the common good rather than on judging the morality of individual actions. At this social action level confronted by legislators and policymakers, the principles of *justice* and *beneficence* weigh more heavily. An individual can interpret an action as being unethical according to his or her personal values, but that does not necessarily mean that the law should penalize the action, unless by doing so, it protects the common good and responds to the principle of *justice.* A parliamentarian who has the personal moral conviction that abortion should be accepted only in very limited situations may vote in favor of the decriminalization of abortion because the legislation is necessary to protect the health of the population. This is, in fact, what many parliamentarians or judges in developed and developing countries have chosen to do when voting, against their personal religious beliefs, to liberalize abortion laws.

Respect for Persons

The principle of *respect for persons,* which is based on the recognition of the right and ability of the individual to become informed and make responsible decisions, favors a woman's right as a full moral agent to decide in conscience to continue or terminate her pregnancy. At the same time, it categorically rejects the notion that a woman can be pressured or forced to terminate her pregnancy. It also means that nobody can be forced to provide abortion services against his or her conscience.

Since respect for individual freedom can be curtailed only to prevent harm to another person, there is a need to establish whether the fertilized egg, the embryo, or the fetus fully qualifies as a person and therefore merits the same respect as the pregnant woman. The progressive development process from one cell, the zygote, to a newborn baby has a parallel in philosophical reflections and legislation from antiquity to today.

Most people seem to agree that the rights of a developing individual increase along with that development, even after birth. In contrast, there are those who argue that the first cell, the zygote, has full moral rights equal to those of an adult. We have to accept that it would probably be impossible to define to everyone's satisfaction, when the existence of another person, with rights equal to those of the woman who carries the pregnancy, begins. Thus, even for those who agree that rights increase with development, the most difficult ethical dilemma is how to decide at which stage of development the fetus acquires legal and moral rights that allow the woman's right to self-determination to be challenged. Some contend that a woman has the right to total autonomy over her body until she has reached full term. We believe that at present there is a general consensus that infanticide is unacceptable. Thus, by analogy, it is difficult to accept the intentional death of a healthy fetus near the end of pregnancy except in the very few cases in which there is no other way to save the woman's life.

For many people, during the first twelve weeks of pregnancy, the existence of the embryo or fetus is not the commanding moral issue. For others, the fetus acquires full moral status after twenty-two weeks when it reaches viability (when it is capable, with appropriate care, of independent life outside the woman's body). Still other markers—such as the woman's perception of fetal movements, or quickening—have a psychological impact on people's view of the acceptability of abortion. Again, although there is no doubt that respect for the fetus increases as gestation progresses, there is no universally accepted gestational age at which the fetus gains full moral recognition.

As we have seen, WHO has set the limit for viability at twenty-two completed weeks of gestation, or a fetus that weighs 500 grams (WHO, 1977). Below this limit, the termination of pregnancy is considered an abortion; after this limit, it becomes a premature birth. The capacity of the fetus to survive outside the woman's body, which defines viability, is a most important distinction in medicine. It determines whether the medical team is responsible for the health of one or two individuals. In the case of an abortion, where the embryo or the fetus is not viable, the product of the reproductive process must be treated with respect, but futile medical attempts to keep the fetus alive must be avoided. The only concern must be the well-being of the woman. After the fetus attains viability, the situation changes: in this case the medical team faces a premature birth that requires all efforts to be directed at protecting the health of both the mother and the fetus, and later the newborn. The exception is the fetus and newborn who is so severely malformed that attempts at survival will also be futile

The various religions take different positions regarding the balance between respect for women as persons and the emergence of the moral value of the fetus. Even the Catholic Church recognizes the problem, explaining that full respect as a person is advisable from the moment of fertilization, because *it is impossible to pinpoint the moment at which a new person exists* (Pérez Aguirre, 2000). In contrast, the Jewish religion traditionally recognizes only the newborn as having developed the full rights of a person. Other religions and schools of thought within religions accept that the fetus acquires full moral value at different gestational ages between these two extremes. This sense of progressive rights is also reflected in present and past abortion legislation, with penalties being more liberal in early pregnancy and increasing in severity as the pregnancy advances.

Even if we accept that the termination of a pregnancy affects two persons with equal rights, this question persists: Which of the two should have priority? The question is particularly relevant when pregnancy threatens the woman's health or life and a choice must be made between the fetus and the woman. Preference for the woman is almost unanimous, even in the Catholic Church, which (by applying the rule of double effect) allows indirect abortion under two specific circumstances: ectopic pregnancy and cancer of the genital organs coexisting with pregnancy (see Chapter 8).

Conversely, the assumption that a woman can be pressured or forced to interrupt her pregnancy is an equal transgression against the ethical principle of *respect for persons.* Sometimes the pressure is less evident (but no less unacceptable), as in the case of a woman who expresses her desire to abort, obtains the support of her partner and family, but later reconsiders and reverses her decision. Partner and family will act unethically if they try to convince her to maintain her earlier decision and exert subtle or not-so-subtle pressure towards that end. A similar situation may exist when a fetus is diagnosed as having severe malformations incompatible with life. The woman has the right to decide to terminate the pregnancy, but she also has the right to choose to continue the pregnancy to term to see the baby before his or her death. It would be unethical on the part of the physician or other staff to try to persuade her either to continue the pregnancy or to abort. Their counseling should be limited to an objective account of the true condition of the fetus and the fetus's prognosis at birth.

Finally, the principle of *respect for persons* also implies that nobody can be forced to provide abortion services against his or her conscience (Cook and Dickens, 1999; Schenker and Cain, 1999). Nevertheless, a serious moral dilemma arises when the health provider who refuses to perform an abortion on the grounds of conscience is the only medical professional accessible to the pregnant woman, particularly if the abortion would save her life. Another unethical practice that we have occasionally observed in countries where abortion is legal under limited circumstances is for doctors who practice illegal abortions in their private practice (for which they are paid on a case-by-case basis) to claim conscientious objection in order to avoid having to perform legal abortions in public hospitals (where they are salaried).

Nonmaleficence/Beneficence

The application of the principles of *nonmaleficence* and *beneficence* to abortion has several implications. Both principles require opposing restrictions to the accessibility of abortion services that can provide legal terminations with a maximum of safety. These restrictions can take the form of (1) the establishment of excessive procedural barriers to legal abortions (as happens sometimes in cases of rape) or (2) physical prevention of access to these services. The application of these principles also implies that the person who performs an abortion should be penalized if he or she does so without the required knowledge and/or the basic technical resources to prevent unnecessary risk of harm to the woman.

Furthermore, global experience shows that not only have countries with laws that seriously restrict abortions failed to decrease the total number of pregnancy terminations; they have, instead, increased the number of abortions performed under unsafe conditions. The consequence has been greater maternal morbidity and mortality and increased death and illness among surviving children of the women who die from unsafe abortions (Buckshee, 1997). In other words, countries with restrictive abortion legislation violate the principles of *nonmaleficence* by maximizing harm to women and society.

The principle of *nonmaleficence* can also be applied to the ethical discussion regarding the gestational age at which pregnancy termination should be accepted. Looking at this problem from a medical perspective, in which the intention is to protect women's health and rights while avoiding a paternalistic attitude, there is little doubt that the earlier the prevention of the birth of an unwanted child is carried out, the better it is for the woman. There is a continuum that starts with avoiding the undesired or unprotected sexual act. Once this has taken place, there is the possibility of emergency contraception to prevent pregnancy. After delayed menstruation, the earlier the abortion can be performed, the lower the risk of psychological and physical trauma for the woman (Brazelton and Cramer, 1990). It is well documented that the later a pregnancy is terminated, the higher the risk to the woman; second-trimester abortions, for example, carry greater risk of medical complications than do earlier pregnancy terminations (Atrash et al., 1987; Lawson et al., 1994).

The question of the woman's increasing psychological attachment to the fetus is less often considered, although its existence is widely accepted by psychologists who deal with this issue (Lumley, 1980; Brazelton and Cramer, 1990). Between fourteen and twenty weeks of pregnancy, women start to feel fetal movement. This first expression of the physical presence of a new being has a dramatic impact on most women, signaling an interchange between the woman and the fetus that ignites a process of emotional interrelation that—especially for those women who want to have a baby—can last forever (Brazelton and Cramer, 1990). Clearly, to have an abortion after fetal movements are perceived exponentially increases the psychological dilemma of pregnancy termination and, for many women, makes the decision even more difficult. Thus, applying the principle of nonmaleficence, there may be a point in time after which the psychological and physical consequences of pregnancy termination may be more detrimental to a woman's well-being than the birth of an unwanted child.

The problem can also be viewed from a different perspective: Why should a woman who suspects she may be pregnant but has no intention of continuing with the pregnancy have to wait until pregnancy is confirmed by clinical or laboratory means in order to have a vacuum aspiration? Evacuation of the uterine content as soon as there is a delay in menstruation is called menstrual regulation. Although in about 80 percent of these cases, pregnancy is present, unconfirmed pregnancy allows reasonable doubt as to whether the procedure constitutes an abortion. Women have the right to know whether or not they are pregnant and the right not to be exposed to the admittedly very small risk of a menstrual regulation they may not need. However, women also have the right to request the procedure without pregnancy testing if they do not wish to know the result. For many women, it is desirable to act within the possibility that what they experienced was the return of a delayed menstruation rather than a terminated pregnancy (Nations et al., 1997).

When menstrual regulation is requested, the professional dilemma for the physician is whether it is ethical to perform the procedure without having made a diagnosis. If the physician lacks laboratory support, there is no good reason to have the woman wait until the pregnancy is clinically confirmed. Even if the physician makes the diagnosis of pregnancy, clinically or through laboratory analysis, he or she has no obligation to disclose it to the patient if the woman has asked not to be told.

Justice

The principle of *justice* serves to enrich the application of the previous principles. Specifically, it forces us not to ignore the fact that the most deprived sectors of society are those whose members really suffer the negative effects of restrictive abortion legislation. Women who are at the lower end of the socioeconomic ladder suffer the rigor of the law and the complications of high-risk abortions. Women in better socioeconomic circumstances frequently obtain illegal but safe abortions. Moreover, restrictive legislation has always penalized the woman but only rarely penalizes the man, who not only shares responsibility for the unwanted pregnancy but also frequently either pressures the woman to abort or creates the circumstances that lead her to choose to do so (Casas, 1996). In other words, in practice, restrictive legislation violates the principle of justice regarding equity with respect to gender and socioeconomic status.

Another ethical problem with restrictive legislation is that it does not respect freedom of religious beliefs, given the great diversity among and within different faiths regarding abortion. The corollary of the freedom to preach and practice a faith is the freedom of others not to be obliged to accept the moral impositions of a religion they do not follow. This was the unanimous conclusion of the meeting of theologians in Genval in 1994 and confirmed in Chiang Mai in 2004, as described in the previous chapter. Participants in those meetings also concluded that decriminalizing abortion is a minimum response for protecting the life and health of women at risk (Park Ridge Center, 1994; Center for Health and Social Policy, 2004). Accordingly, if we look at the problem from the perspective of religious freedom, the concept that restrictive abortion legislation violates the principle of *justice* is further reinforced.

The Ethical Dilemma for Gynecologists/Obstetricians

In any discussion of ethical values with respect to abortion, it is pertinent to include the official ethical views of the medical specialists who deal professionally with these issues. Gynecologists and obstetricians are organized, at national and regional levels, in scientific associations that are affiliated with FIGO. One of FIGO's permanent bodies, the Committee for the Study of Ethical Aspects of Human Reproduction and the Health of Women (note that both authors of this book have been members of this committee), analyzed the complex moral dilemma of induced abortion during three of its sessions (May 1997, March 1998, and September 1998). The guidelines agreed upon by the committee ask for increased efforts to prevent unintended pregnancies, recognizing the right of women to choose whether or not to reproduce. They further state, "Providing the process of properly informed consent has been carried out, a woman's right to autonomy, combined with the need to prevent unsafe abortion, justifies the provision of safe abortion." In summary, the committee recommended that "after appropriate counseling, a woman had the right to have access to medical or surgical induced abortion, and that the health care service had an obligation to provide such services as safely as possible" (Schenker and Cain, 1999, p. 320).

These guidelines were published by FIGO with the caution (applicable to all agreements of the committee) that they were "not intended to reflect an official position of FIGO, but to provide material for consideration and debate about these ethical aspects of [the organization's] discipline for member organizations and their constituent membership" (Schenker and Cain, 1999, p. 317). Nevertheless, in September 2000, the General Assembly of FIGO unanimously adopted these guidelines as the official policy of the organization. FIGO had not adopted ethical guidelines as a policy since the creation of the committee in 1985. This was a demonstration of the profession's worldwide commitment to decreasing the suffering of women from abortion. Later evaluation showed that these ethical guidelines have been, in general, well accepted in different countries, including colleagues from countries with restrictive abortion laws (McKay, Rogo, and Dixon, 2001).

Our Reflections on Ethical Values
Concerning Abortion

Our analysis, which attempts a balanced application of the four bioethical principles to the problem of induced abortion, has led us to the following conclusions:

1. During the first twelve weeks of pregnancy, the principle of *autonomy* should be given priority, allowing women to decide to abort for a wide range of reasons. We make this distinction in recognition that the rights of the embryo/fetus increase with the length of pregnancy, as does the risk of the procedure to the woman. We recognize that twelve weeks is an arbitrary figure, but it can be justified because it marks (a) the highest gestational age that allows low-risk pregnancy termination and (b) some important anatomical and physiological changes in fetal development, such as the beginning of brain life (Sass, 1994).

2. Abortion beyond twelve weeks of gestation should be accepted only with a strong justification. The definition of *strong justification* depends on the circumstances, including the values of the local culture. We believe that risk to women's life, very severe fetal malformation, and pregnancy as a result of rape or incest should be included in this category.

3. After twenty-two weeks (when the fetus is viable), a termination of pregnancy will be a premature birth rather than an abortion; accordingly, efforts should be made to postpone the procedure in order to achieve the greatest possible maturity and chance of survival for the fetus without exposing the woman's health to excessive risk. Termination of pregnancy beyond twenty-two weeks of gestation should be permitted when it threatens the life of the woman or when current technology identifies a severe fetal malformation that is incompatible with life outside the uterus. Women pregnant with a malformed fetus should not, however, be pressured to abort if they wish to carry the pregnancy to term.

We believe that these conclusions can provide an ethical basis on which to pursue a dialogue aimed at achieving a social consensus on abortion as will be discussed further in the last part of this book.

10
Values as Reflected in the Law

Laws are the instruments used by governments to provide the basis for deciding when an act is permitted or when it should be penalized. However, laws do not always fulfill their intended purpose: the regulation of social and personal behavior. Their effectiveness depends on how well they respond to the values of the community in which they are applied. Legal systems work best when they are based on values that reflect a social consensus; laws that lack substantial social support not only are rarely enforced but also discredit the legal system. This is the case with many laws that attempt to regulate sexuality, reproduction, and (particularly) abortion. If the restrictive abortion laws that prevail in many developing countries were truly enforced, there would never be sufficient room in the jails to receive all the offenders.

The habitual defiance of restrictive abortion laws does not, however, eliminate their impact on the attitude of providers and society at large. As we have already seen in previous chapters, restrictive laws limit access to safe abortion, exponentially increasing the consequences of unsafe procedures. In order to help inform the public about the legal aspects of the abortion debate, therefore, it is necessary to review the differences between abortion laws in different regions. We start by describing the various legal systems as they relate to the application of abortion laws, reviewing the evolution of these laws during the past two centuries. We also provide some global statistical information about the legality of abortion, with a focus on concepts that can help clarify the debate. Finally, we briefly review some of the widely accepted international conventions with respect to the social regulation of abortion.

Legal Systems

Currently, most countries can be broadly categorized within one of three major types of legal systems: civil law, common law, and Islamic law (United Nations, 2001a, 2001b, 2002).

1. The civil law system, which has its origin in Roman law and in the Napoleonic Code (dated 1810), is based on codified laws devoted to specific topics. This system serves as a general guide to the proper conduct of individuals and as a means of preserving justice and morality in society as a whole. Placing an emphasis on social responsibility, the rights of the person are viewed within their social context rather than as separate and inalienable entitlements of individuals. Interpretation by judges plays a relatively minor role in shaping the law.

2. The common law system, which follows the traditional English model, is based on court determinations made by judges. Written laws emphasize crime and punishment for "unlawful" actions; "lawful" actions are, in contrast, unwritten and interpretable by the courts. Law is viewed primarily as a means of resolving disputes among individuals. This system emphasizes principles of self-reliance and individual rights, such as property rights and freedom of contract, more than the order and welfare of society. Law is changed not primarily by government action but through the development of a body of court decisions that reflect evolving judicial interpretation as social conditions change. Although statutes are enacted, the common law system offers judges a much greater judicial leeway than the civil law system, giving the law more flexibility.

3. Islamic law, known as *Shariah,* differs in that its conception is bound to religion. Law under Islam is based primarily on the text of the Koran, the holy book of Islam, and the *sunnah,* the collection of acts and statements made by the prophet Mohammed, which are considered a guide for human conduct. Therefore, Islamic law is for the most part considered to have been predetermined; hence set, permanent, and invariable except with respect to issues and situations, such as abortion, that are not specifically encountered in the Koran and *sunnah.* In these cases, Islamic jurists engage in interpretation, using deductive or analogical reasoning to seek consensus, which varies greatly from one Islamic legal school to another.

The civil law system is followed in virtually all of Europe, Latin America, non-Anglophone African countries, most former Soviet republics, Japan, and Turkey. The common law system operates in the United Kingdom and in most of the former colonies of the British Empire. Islamic law is followed in most of the Muslim countries in Asia and Africa.

Legal Systems and Abortion

As described above, the law can be more or less explicit according to the legal system adopted. Even when laws are very explicit, some person or system must interpret their application in each particular case. As we have seen, the freedom of the judges and courts to interpret the law is greatest under the common law system.

Clearly, the more explicitly that laws and regulations are written, the more easily and rigidly they are applied. This legal attribute acquires particular relevance with respect to abortion, because the explicit nature of a law strongly influences the attitude of the professional who bears responsibility for carrying out the termination of a pregnancy. In many countries, although abortion is considered a crime according to legislation, the same laws establish that neither the woman nor the practitioner is condemned if certain conditions are present. In other words, abortion is always a crime and physicians who perform the abortion and the women who abort can be prosecuted, but they will not be condemned if these exceptional circumstances are present. For a health professional, there is a great difference between legislation that gives a clear mandate with respect to what she or he can legally do, and legislation that merely provides a loophole for a legal defense if the individual is faced with a trial.

The Napoleonic Code, which is the paradigm of the civil law system, punished abortion with imprisonment, but it was understood that abortion could be performed to save the life of the pregnant woman. France made this exception explicit in 1939 and passed remarkably liberal abortion legislation in 1979.

English law traditionally considered abortion an offense but defined pregnancy as beginning at quickening. In 1803 abortion before quickening also became a criminal offense, but it was less severely punished than post-quickening abortion. Abortions performed on the grounds that they were necessary to save the woman's life were interpreted as valid exceptions. In 1967 Great Britain adopted its Abortion Act, which sets forth broad justifications for abortion (e.g., the health of the woman, fetal impairment, and socioeconomic considerations). The 1967 Abortion Act was followed by similar legislation in some commonwealth nations, including India and Zambia (Cook and Dickens, 1999).

In contrast to civil and common law systems, classic Islamic law punishes abortion with payment of a sum of money to the relatives of the fetus. The amount of payment increases according to the length of the pregnancy at the time of its termination. National abortion laws in Islamic countries vary from among the most liberal to among the most restrictive; in every case, however, abortion to save a woman's life—regardless of gestational age of the fetus—is allowed.

The Legality of Abortion Around the World

Before 1800, abortion was not a major legal issue, and it was not until the nineteenth century that restrictive abortion laws proliferated in Europe. It is speculated that the restrictive laws were intended to reduce the increasing number of abortions and the resultant maternal deaths attributed to the high-risk procedures used at the time. It was only natural that the same laws were extended to European colonies in other continents, which maintained the legislation after independence.

Since the 1960s, as abortion procedures have become safer and the preference for small families has increased in the developed countries, the trend has been to decriminalize abortion or at least to liberalize the conditions under which it is considered legal, particularly during early pregnancy. This liberalization of abortion laws has begun later in developing countries, where there has been a truly significant fall in fertility rates only in recent decades. This trend was more in evidence between 1985 and 1997, when abortion laws were liberalized in ten developed and nine developing countries with populations of more than one million people each (Alan Guttmacher Institute, 1999). Although the trend continues to this day, abortion laws in developing countries remain relatively restrictive.

A recent review of this subject (Center for Reproductive Rights, 2003), which includes countries or territories with more than one million inhabitants each, shows that 64.5 percent of the world's population lives in eighty-eight countries or territories where the law permits abortion under a wide range of circumstances. In all of these countries and territories, abortion is allowed to save the life or preserve the health of the pregnant woman. In addition, in twenty of these countries, representing three percent of the world's population, the law explicitly permits abortion to preserve the woman's mental health. In another fourteen countries, which make up 21 percent of the population, the procedure is also allowed for socioeconomic reasons, and in the remaining fifty-four countries, constituting 40.5 percent of the population, no justification for abortion is required during at least the first twelve weeks of pregnancy. For the most part, these countries in which abortion is legal in a wide range of circumstances usually establish some other conditions in addition to gestational age. They specify, for example, necessary qualifications for those who are allowed to perform abortions and required conditions for facilities in which abortions can be performed. Some require informed consent, counseling, and waiting periods (Allan Guttmacher Institute, 1999).

In contrast, abortion is much more restricted in 107 countries, representing 36 percent of the world's population. In 33 of them, constituting 10 percent of the population, abortion is permitted only to save the life of or preserve the health of the woman. In the remaining 74 countries, making up 26 percent of the world's population, abortion is allowed only to save the life of the woman or (in the case of two of these countries) not at all (Center for Reproductive Rights, 2003).

The Population Division of the United Nations reviewed abortion policies up to 1999, covering 193 countries irrespective of their size and population. The result of this review is summarized in Table 10.1.

The first line of the table indicates that most, but not all countries permit abortion to save the woman's life. Moreover, it can be argued that there is no exception: one of the countries that does not allow abortion under any circumstances is the Holy See, a territory whose population

Table 10.1. Circumstances under which abortion is permitted in 193 countries. Source: United Nations, Population Division, New York, 1999.

Circumstance	Developed Countries (48)		Developing Countries (145)		All Countries (193)	
	Number	%	Number	%	Number	%
Preservation of the woman's life	46	(96)	143	(99)	189	(98)
Preservation of physical health	42	(88)	80	(55)	122	(63)
Preservation of mental health	41	(85)	79	(54)	120	(62)
Rape or incest	39	(81)	44	(30)	83	(43)
Fetal impairment	39	(81)	37	(26)	76	(39)
Socioeconomic concerns	36	(75)	27	(19)	63	(33)
Upon request	31	(65)	21	(14)	52	(27)

presumably lacks this type of moral dilemma. In the three other countries that do not allow abortion under any circumstances (Chile, El Salvador, and Malta), "it is not clear . . . whether a defense of necessity might be allowed to justify an abortion performed to save the life of the woman" (United Nations, 1999, n. 59).

Penal codes have general provisions that allow illegal acts to be performed without punishment when they are necessary to preserve a good. In these three countries, this general provision could be evoked in the legal defense of an abortion trial. We, the authors of this book, can testify that at least in Chile and to a lesser degree in El Salvador, abortions to treat ectopic pregnancies or cancer of the genital tract of the pregnant woman are performed by the medical profession with no legal repercussions.

In addition, the table indicates that abortion laws tend to be more restrictive in the less developed regions of the world than in the developed countries. While the laws in 65 percent of developed countries allow abortion under all of the circumstances listed in Table 10.1, only 14 percent of developing countries have laws that are equally permissive. The UN Population Division study also showed regional differences among developing countries. Their laws allow abortion under all circumstances considered, as follows: in 35.5 percent of the countries located in Asia (sixteen out of forty-five) but in only 6 percent of those located either in Africa (three out of fifty-three: Cape Verde, South Africa, and Tunisia) or in Latin America and the Caribbean (two out of thirty-three: Cuba and Guyana). None of the fourteen developing countries located in Oceania has such liberal abortion laws.

A further complication is that in federal countries, such as Mexico, laws on abortion may differ among states and state law may differ from federal law. It is outside the scope of this book to attempt to analyze this wide variety of situations.

Human Rights Declarations and Conventions

Although the term *human rights* is most commonly understood to connote universal moral values, it has been used with various other meanings in the abortion debate. This chapter refers to human rights in a more limited and precise sense, as *rights that governments have collectively recognized as inherent to human dignity*, which they are therefore obligated to respect in their legislation and in the application of their laws.

The concept of basic or fundamental human rights that should be protected by all countries was first recognized by the governments of the world in 1948, when the United Nations adopted the Universal Declaration of Human Rights. This document and subsequent declarations by the international community reflect an official consensus reached by representatives of the countries of the world in international meetings convened to determine how societies should behave.

The drafting of an international declaration is followed by a long process before it can become a binding legal obligation for any country. After representatives attending an international conference sign a declaration, it must be officially signed by the represented nations, which frequently note explicit reservations about specific points. Declarations, however, are not legally binding documents. Although these documents are mere promises of hope, they reflect an important first step toward the assumption of legal obligations and are the basis on which legally binding treaties are subsequently negotiated.

Treaties, called conventions or covenants, are first adopted by the United Nations with the vote of the countries' official representatives, who may again at this time note reservations about specific points.

Finally, for these treaties to become part of national law, countries must *ratify* or *accede to* them through their usual legislative procedures, generally by parliamentary action. In doing so, nations may note reservations, which they can later eliminate by a new parliamentary action. Countries are accountable to the international community for honoring treaties that they have ratified (Panos Health and Reproductive Health Reports, 1998).

By their very nature and origin, human rights are defined in general terms and cannot be expected to operate in absolute terms because they will be often in conflict with each other. Even if they do not conflict, they must be interpreted according to the particular circumstances in question. Balancing rights in conflict and interpreting their application in the absence of a global government must be left to the discretion of the government of each individual country.

In view of these circumstances, treaties have established international independent supervisory bodies with specific mechanisms and authority (according to each treaty) to monitor and encourage compliance. For example, the Convention on the Elimination of All Forms of Discrimination against Women (the Women's Convention) established the Committee on the Elimination of All Forms of Discrimination Against Women (CEDAW), which analyzes and comments on periodic reports that governments submit about their compliance with the treaty. Many countries have similarly entered into binding *regional* human rights treaties, such as the Inter-American Convention on the Prevention and Punishment of Violence against Women [the Belém do Para Convention].

In spite of their many limitations, internationally sanctioned human rights represent important social progress: they provide a mechanism that allows countries to agree on basic universal values and to give moral support to the complaints of the oppressed. However, as Michael Ignatieff has pointed out: "The rights language states that all human beings belong at the table in the essential conversation about how we should treat each other. But once this universal right to speak and be heard is granted, there is bound to be . . . conflict, deliberation, argument, and contention. We need to stop thinking of human rights as trumps and begin thinking of them as part of a language that creates the basis for deliberation. In this argument, the ground we share may actually be quite limited; not much more than the basic intuition that what is pain and humiliation for you is bound to be pain and humiliation for me. But this is already something. In such a future, shared among equals, rights are not the universal credo of a global society, not a secular religion, but something much more limited and yet just as valuable: the shared vocabulary from which our arguments can begin, and the bare human minimum from which differing ideas of human flourishing can take root" (Ignatieff, 2001).

Abortion Laws and Human Rights

Abortion creates a tension between two human rights: the right to life of the embryo or fetus and the autonomy of the pregnant women (a basic component of the right to freedom). Since there is no hierarchical order of human rights, when they are in conflict, an individual interpretation is required to enable their application (Cook, 2000). This has been recognized by UN member states in their consensus that human rights are interdependent, indivisible, and integral (United Nations, 1993). UN member states have further agreed (United Nations, 1995b) that women's human rights include their entitlement to control over and free and responsible decision making with respect to matters related to their sexuality—including sexual and reproductive health—without coercion, discrimination, or violence. Relationships where women and men are on equal terms in matters of sexual relations and reproduction include full respect for the integrity of the person and require mutual respect, consent, and shared responsibility for sexual behavior and its consequences.

In addition, the Beijing Platform for Action expressly condemned sexual slavery, rape, sexual abuse, and forced pregnancy, including both forced initiation of pregnancy and forced continuation of pregnancy. These declarations put into question restrictive abortion laws that force women to continue pregnancies against their will.

Furthermore, the 187 governments that adopted the Beijing Platform committed to consider "reviewing laws containing punitive measures against women who have undergone illegal abortions" (United Nations, 1995b, para. 106 item k).

As we have seen, UN committees that monitor states' compliance with human rights resolutions notify governments (usually by response to the countries' official reports) when they have failed to fulfill their obligations. For example, in 1996 the UN Human Rights Committee's response to the Report of the Government of Peru addressed the human rights of women, including the rights denied them by the criminal abortion law of Peru. The committee expressed concern that abortion incurs a criminal penalty even if the woman is pregnant as a result of rape and that unsafe abortion is the main cause of maternal mortality. The committee found that, contrary to Article 7 of the International Covenant on Civil and Political Rights, the criminal law subjected women to inhumane treatment (Cook, 2000).

Similarly, CEDAW has commented on the reports of several countries. In 1997, after reviewing the report from Morocco, the committee expressed concern about the high rate of maternal mortality, the high number of unintended births, the lack of access to safe abortions, and the need for further reproductive and sexual health services, including family planning. It considered Turkey's legal requirement that a woman's husband authorize her abortion a violation of her right, under the convention, to equality under the law (Cook, 2000).

Human rights arguments are also used at the national level to justify changes in governments' laws. For example, in 1988 the Supreme Court of Canada declared restrictive abortion laws unconstitutional because they denied women's fundamental rights. Canada's chief justice observed that forcing a woman, by threat of criminal sanction, to carry a fetus to term unless she meets certain criteria unrelated to her own priorities and aspirations is a profound interference with a woman's body and thus a violation of the security of that person (Cook, 2000).

Another example is South Africa's 1996 Choice on Termination of

Pregnancy Act, which further liberalized abortion legislation in that country. The preamble explains that the legislation was proposed for the advancement of human rights and freedoms that underscore a democratic South Africa. The Act, which repeals previous legislation, promotes reproductive rights and extends freedom of choice by affording every woman the right to decide whether to undergo an early, safe, and legal termination of pregnancy according to her individual beliefs (paragraph 7). The Act legalizes abortion upon a woman's request up to twelve weeks of pregnancy; abortions up to twenty weeks on grounds of risk to physical or mental health, socioeconomic concerns, and rape or incest; and after twenty weeks on grounds of risk to the woman's life or risk of severe fetal malformation. Third-party authorizations for married women or minors are not required under any circumstances (Cook, 2000).

Interestingly, a South African association sued the minister of health and sought a judicial declaration of the unconstitutionality of the 1996 Act. The association argued that the life of a human being begins at conception and is therefore protected by section 11 of the 1996 South African Constitution, which states that everyone has the right to life. The judge refused the declaration on the grounds that the term *everyone* is a legal alternative to the expression *every person* and that personhood historically commences only at live birth. The judge found it unnecessary to address the claim that the biological beginning of human life is at conception, since the beginning of human life does not, in any case, mark the beginning of a legal person. He observed, "The question is not whether a conceptus is human but whether it should be given the same legal protection as you and me" (Cook, 2000, p. 85).

In contrast, in 1997 the Constitutional Tribunal of Poland ruled that a liberalized abortion law approved the previous year was incompatible with constitutional rights intended to protect human life in every phase of its development, starting at conception. The tribunal found that it was its constitutionally imposed duty to protect motherhood and the family and that the constitutional interests of an unborn human life could not be decided by vague criteria of women's conditions or situations, particularly when such conditions or situations were to be determined, as the previous year's law had provided, by women themselves. Thus, challenging women's capacity to act as moral agents, abortion on demand or for socioeconomic reasons was forbidden. Abortion remained legal on grounds of preservation of the life of or the health of the woman (without distinguishing between physical and mental health), rape or incest, and fetal impairment. Nevertheless, access to abortion in Poland has, in practice, become quite restricted, regardless of the justification (Cook, 2000).

General Conclusion on Abortion and the Law

National laws treat abortion in many different ways and allow for abortion under a variety of circumstances. The global consensus exists, however, that abortion must be legal to save the life of the woman. Moreover, there is a clear trend, no longer limited to developed countries, toward the liberalization of abortion laws. Human rights arguments, although used both for and against the liberalization of abortion laws, are applied predominantly and increasingly for the former purpose.

In our view, this changing panorama of the legality of abortion reflects a growing international consensus not only that restrictive abortion laws are ineffective in decreasing the number of abortions but also that they trigger tragic social and public health consequences.

PART III

Improving the Situation

11
How to Decrease
the Number of Abortions

Legal and Moral Prohibition

Despite global evidence to the contrary, many political and religious leaders and rank-and-file promoters of the pro-life movement continue to believe that the best way to reduce the number of abortions is through legal and moral prohibition.

The idea behind the prohibition of abortion and the condemnation and penalization of women who abort is that women would decide to let an unwanted pregnancy continue if the price they had to pay for aborting were raised to intolerable heights. Implicit in this idea is the concept that (1) these women have other viable alternatives and (2) in an environment where abortion is broadly accepted, the toll of abortion is too low.

The dilemma for a woman with an unwanted pregnancy is the choice between an abortion and an unwanted baby. The alternative in many countries is carrying the pregnancy to term, with the possibility of giving the child up for adoption after delivery. Some women may prefer or be obliged by circumstances to accept this alternative: for example, they may be unable to pay the fee charged by the abortionist, self-abortion may have failed, or they may have reached the decision to abort too late in the pregnancy.

In some cases where the attempt to abort fails, the woman may decide to keep her child. Sometimes the result will be a good mother-child relationship and a happy ending. The evidence, however, is that an unwanted pregnancy taken to term is much more likely to end with a troubled child and an ill-adapted adult than would be the case when the child was wanted from the beginning (Matejcek, Dytrych, and Schüller, 1985; David et al., 1988). In other words, under certain circumstances the obstacles that society imposes to impede abortion may work, but the end result will not necessarily be positive.

What is very clear is that the most severe restrictions and strict enforcement of anti-abortion laws, including the incarceration of women who have induced abortions, are not at all efficient in reducing the number of abortions. Moreover, there is strong evidence that decidedly liberal abortion laws, which provide easy access to pregnancy termination, do not necessarily lead to a high incidence of abortion.

Countries in Latin America, where abortion is severely restricted or totally prohibited, have relatively high incidences of abortion, ranging from thirty-five to fifty abortions per thousand women of childbearing age per year (Singh and Wulf, 1994). These rates are five to ten times greater than in western European countries, such as the Netherlands or Germany, where abortion is broadly permitted and easily accessible (Singh and Wulf, 1994; Henshaw, Singh, and Haas, 1999). The problem is that restrictive abortion laws do not address the source of the matter: the occurrence of unwanted pregnancy. A number of conditions in the Netherlands that do not exist in the Latin American countries (see the later discussion under "Prevention of Unwanted Pregnancy") explain the difference in the abortion rates (Ketting and Visser, 1994).

In order to identify which actions can reduce abortion, it is important to recall why women have unwanted pregnancies as we discussed in the first part of this book We have seen that the main determinants of unwanted pregnancy are women's lack of power over their sexual activity; women's lack of education, including inadequate and inaccurate knowledge of contraceptive methods; limited access to effective contraception; and the absence of social support for pregnant women and their children. As long as these conditions exist, a large number of unwanted pregnancies will occur, and, despite legal, moral, or religious prohibitions and sanctions, most will result in abortion.

This is precisely the situation for the majority of Latin American and African women. Only recently has there been improvement in access to contraceptive methods in some countries, but this progress is outweighed by other restrictions that remain. Clearly, the high abortion rate reflects an increased incidence of unwanted pregnancy, which—as we have seen—results from imposed, unprotected sex; limited knowledge of contraception; unreliable access to fertility regulation methods; and lack of social support.

The response of many political and religious leaders in countries with restrictive laws is to do nothing or to oppose interventions that prevent unwanted pregnancy. They try to force women to carry their unwanted pregnancies to term without providing the social support that they and their families need to live with a minimum of dignity, safe from hunger, homelessness, and disease.

Prevention of Unwanted Pregnancies

Every abortion is the result of an unwanted pregnancy. Clearly, therefore, the first strategy for decreasing the number of abortions is to help women avoid pregnancy when they do not want to have a baby. These measures will, in turn, reduce another important social problem: the incidence of unwanted babies (Stille, 2001). Even after unwanted pregnancy has occurred, the number of unwanted babies can be reduced, by providing pregnant women with the social support they need to continue the pregnancy without undue distress and to carry out their pre-pregnancy plans for the future. Admittedly, however, this strategy is both expensive and difficult to achieve with any success.

Global experience drives the preference for prevention of unwanted pregnancy as the primary strategy for decreasing the number of abortions. The low abortion rate in the Netherlands coincides with conditions that favor the prevention of unintended pregnancies. The high incidence of abortion in Latin America and eastern Europe corresponds to limited access to effective means of preventing unwanted pregnancies. (Hardy et al., 1990; Alvarez, 1992; Ketting and Visser, 1994).

Contraceptive Services and the Reduction of Unwanted Pregnancies

As we have seen, the 1994 ICPD affirmed the human rights of women with respect to reproductive and sexual health. On the subject of abortion, the conference participants recognized unsafe abortion as a major public health concern and pledged their commitment to reducing the need for abortion "through expanded and improved family planning services" (United Nations, 1995a, p. 44).

This statement seems to indicate that the governments of the world, present at the Cairo Conference, understood that improving family planning services was the *intervention* likely to be most effective in reducing unwanted pregnancies and abortions, a conviction based on the success of programs aimed at making contraceptive information and services accessible to women.

Global experience indicates that there is an interval between the increase in access to knowledge and contraception and the decrease in the number of abortions. It appears that societies evolve from a culture of large families with many children to one of fewer children. During the period of rapid reduction in the ideal number of children, there is a parallel rise in the number of abortions. When contraceptive knowledge and services become increasingly available, the prevalence of contraceptive use grows, but the number of abortions does not immediately decrease. It appears that whereas some women shift from abortion to contraception, others move from childbirth to abortion. Only once access to contraceptives and efficiency of service reach an adequate level does the incidence of abortion show a quick downturn.

This process was described in 1969 by Requena, who observed that whereas women in the higher strata of Chilean society were having few children and few abortions and were using contraception, women at a lower socioeconomic level were having few children and more abortions and were less likely to use contraception. Women in the very lowest strata were having more children and fewer abortions and were using contraception minimally. Requena schematically illustrated this process (see Figure 11.1). *

One of the first social interventions specifically aimed at reducing the incidence of abortion was carried out in Chile in the early to mid-1960s. An initial population-based survey was carried out in a working-class community of about twenty thousand people on the outskirts of Santiago. Knowledge and use of contraceptive methods and pregnancy history were assessed in a representative sample of women in the community.

The intervention consisted of adding family planning care to the services already being provided at the maternal and child care public health clinic that served the community. The provision of contraceptive pills, IUDs, and injections was included among the clinic's services. The community organizations were asked to disseminate information on the risks of abortion and the availability of new, safe, effective contraceptive methods at the community health center (Faúndes, Rodrigues-Galant, and Avendaño, 1968). The population-based survey was repeated two and four years after the initiation of the intervention. A dramatic increase

---

*The term pregnancy history refers to a methodology originally designed by Donald Bogue at the Centro Latinoamericano de Demografia (CELADE), widely adopted as a standard means of obtaining information for each month of a woman's reproductive life span by recording whether or not she has been exposed to pregnancy and the consequences of that exposure (Faúndes, Rodrigues-Galant, and Avendaño, 1968).

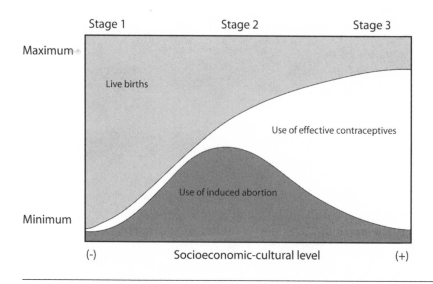

Figure 11.1. Evolution of childbirth, abortion, and contraceptive prevalence by socioeconomic-cultural level. Source: Requena, 1969.

in knowledge about and use of contraceptive methods was observed, with a correspondingly dramatic decrease in the abortion rate (see Figure 11.2) (Faúndes et al., 1971).

Starting in late 1966, a family planning component became an official part of the women's health care program in Chile, providing free contraceptive services to 85 percent of the population through the highly efficient National Health Service (Rosselot et al., 1966). Subsequent evaluations showed a direct correlation between improved access to contraceptives and the dramatic decrease in the number of women with abortion complications who were admitted to public hospitals, replicating at the national level the results of the community study previously described (Maine, 1981; Viel, 1985; Barzelatto, 1986). Figure 11.3 shows the abrupt decrease in the rate of abortion complications in the capital city of Santiago, with no change in the trend of a slowly decreasing birth rate (Barzelatto, 1986).

More recent observations of the correlation between the use of contraceptives and abortion rates in other countries confirm the effectiveness of contraception in reducing the incidence of abortion. An analysis of data from three Latin American countries, compiled by researchers from the Alan Guttmacher Institute during the 1980s and 1990s, showed that Mexico and Colombia followed the same pattern observed in Chile:

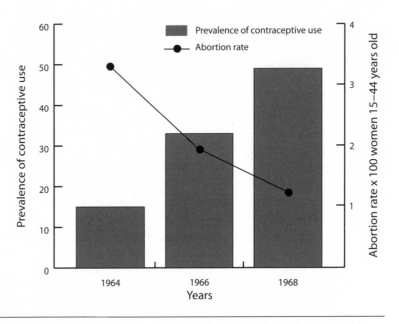

Figure 11.2. Prevalence of contraceptive use and the rate of abortion in San Gregório, Santiago de Chile, 1964 to 1968. Source: Faúndes et al., 1971.

an increase in the number of abortions coinciding with a decrease in the ideal number of children followed by stabilization and later a decrease in the abortion rate as the proportion of women using contraception increased (Singh and Sedgh, 1997). In that study Brazil was the exception, but later data showed that following the rapid increase in the proportion of women who use modern contraceptives, the number of abortion complications attended by the national health service l dropped from about 345,000 in 1992 to 228,000 in 1998 (UNFPA, 1995; Ministério da Saúde do Brasil, 1999).

In a recent analysis carried out by Cicely Marston and John Cleland (2003) in thirteen countries with reliable statistics from different regions of the world, these patterns of contraceptive use and incidence of abortion were confirmed. When the birth rate is stable, the number of abortions decreases as the use of modern contraceptives increases. When there is a rapid decrease in fertility, both abortions and contraceptive use increase simultaneously because contraception alone is not sufficient to control the birth rate at the outset. However, once fertility stabilizes, as contraceptive use grows, induced abortions invariably decline.

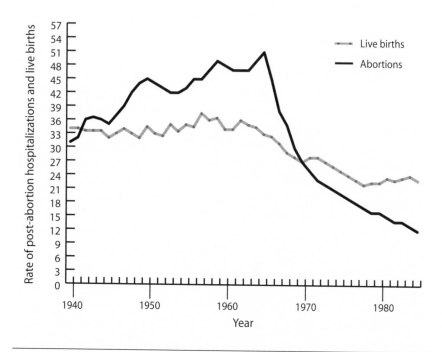

Figure 11.3. Rate of post-abortion hospitalizations per thousand women of childbearing age in Santiago de Chile and crude birth rate per thousand midyear population in Chile, 1940 to 1984. Source: Barzelatto, 1986 to 1989), and the period when it became legal again (post-1989). Source: Stephenson et al., 1992; WHO, 1997.

A look at the countries with the highest abortion rates—Cuba and the nations of eastern Europe—reveals that the common denominator is scarce and undependable access to reliable contraceptive methods (Popov, 1991; Alvarez et al., 1999). Only high-dose pills, outdated non-copper-bearing IUDs, and (to a very limited degree) condoms were available in Cuba, whereas in the Western world and Asia, low-dose pills, copper IUDs, and (to a much greater extent) condoms were available. In general, it appears that in countries with high abortion rates, women perceive abortion as much more accessible than contraception. Th situation is slowly changing but will probably take some time to revert. In Cuba, as better contraceptives have become available in recent years, the abortion rate has decreased approximately 50 percent (Ministerio de Salud Pública de Cuba, 2001).

In contrast, in countries with a low incidence of abortion—below ten per thousand women of childbearing age per year—there is broad knowledge of and easy access to effective contraceptive methods (Ketting and Visser, 1994; Moore, 2000). Although there is also easy access to abortionthe observed behavior indicates that women have an overwhelming preference for the prevention of unwanted pregnancy over pregnancy termination.

Other barriers to the accessibility of contraception, mostly affecting adolescents, are observed in both developed and developing countries. Among the most common impediments are unfriendly or inappropriate delivery systems and cultural values. Adolescents treated for abortion complications in Tanzania were unaware that they had a right to request contraceptive services at the public family planning clinics (Silberschmidt and Rasch, 2001). Belgian adolescents were inhibited by cost, waiting time, and fear of gynecological examination (Peremans et al., 2000). Young women in Missouri and in Bombay, India, mentioned embarrassment as a barrier to the acquisition of condoms (Sable and Libbus, 1998; Roth, Krishnan, and Bunch, 2001). In order to overcome these obstacles, several recent initiatives that target adolescents have introduced innovative techniques that have been successful in increasing condom use (Johns Hopkins Center for Communication Programs, 2001; Underwood et al., 2001).

In summary, most evidence points to the fact that the provision of information and services that allow women to control their fertility greatly reduces unwanted pregnancy and abortion, and global experience has highlighted the most efficient ways to do so.

Increase Women's Power

Many women who have had abortions point to imposed sexual intercourse as the cause of the unintended pregnancy (Kabir, 1989; Mashabala, 1989). Numerous studies carried out in a variety of different cultures have documented that a large proportion of women—most frequently adolescent girls—submit to sexual intercourse against their will (Heise, Pitanguy, and Germain, 1994). It has also been observed that as women become more assertive in challenging traditional gender norms, their bargaining power with respect to protected sex greatly increases (Machel, 2001).

As described in Chapter 5, sex can be imposed on women by several different means, from physical aggression to the cultural acceptance of a male's rights over a woman's body. This involves not only the imposition of unwanted sex but also the imposition of sex under unwanted conditions (for example, when the woman is denied the opportunity to protect herself against unwanted pregnancy and disease). Clearly, a significant number of unwanted pregnancies occur among women who know about and have access to contraception but who, through male abuse of sexual power, do not have the opportunity to use them. One common manifestation of such power is the husband's veto of his wife's contraceptive use (Ezeh, 1993). Removing the requirement for a husband's approval is, accordingly, an effective way to increase the number of women who use contraceptives (Cook and Maine, 1987).

Fortunately the culture of male dominance is not irreversible. Gender equity has greatly advanced in some countries, with certain aspects of the gender power imbalance more resistant than others. Whereas equal pay for equal work is more difficult to achieve, sharing family responsibilities—including fertility control—is increasingly being observed. A fair power balance with respect to sex-related decisions has also been achieved in several developed countries. It is noteworthy that countries with a low incidence of abortion—such as those in western Europe—are also countries with a fairly good gender power balance (Moore, 2000). Furthermore, research in developing countries shows that the model of gender dominance can be shifted through programs that target males during childhood and adolescence (Barker and Lowenstein, 1997).

Improvement of men's awareness of their reproductive responsibility and the importance of sharing power within the relationship depends on the development of effective gender and sex education for adult males as well. Reproductive health programs in developing countries, where the gender power imbalance is greater than in developed countries, rarely pursue such strategies, which could have a great impact on women's access to contraception. The presumption that this is an almost impossible task is not sustained by evidence: A study in India showed that properly informed men were more willing to take additional reproductive responsibility (Balaiah et al., 1999).

The evaluation of sex education programs provide the best evidence that the gender power balance as it relates to sexual activity has the potential for change. The vast majority of studies have shown that sex education programs of adequate duration and methodology that promote responsibility, abstinence, and (for those who are sexually active) protection against pregnancy and disease are effective in reducing pregnancy and abortion (Grunseit et al., 1997; Kirby, 2001). When sex education programs are implemented before sexual activity has begun, they are particularly effective in promoting both abstinence and the use of contraception (Grunseit, 1997).

Sex education does not increase sexual activity or promote early experimentation, as some conservative sectors of society have feared,. In fact, it may encourage adolescents to postpone the initiation of sexual activity and thus reduce the proportion of adolescents who have sexual relations (Dawson, 1986; Pick et al., 1990; Kirby et al., 1993; Sathe, 1994; Grunseit, 1997; Mbizvo et al., 1997, Kirby, 2001).

The promotion of mutual respect and gender power balance through sex education is not enough, however. It is essential for women and girls to have a minimal knowledge of reproductive physiology and sexually transmitted disease. Unfortunately, particularly among young people in some of the developing countries, this knowledge is painfully lacking (Oyediran, Ishola, and Adewuyi, 2002).

Countries with the lowest abortion rates are those that have broad-based, progressive sex education programs in their schools and nearly universal school attendance. The success of the Nordic European countries in reducing the number of teen abortions and teen pregnancies is evidenced by the fact that their teen abortion and pregnancy rates are now among the lowest in the world: Adolescent deliveries are rare, just over five per thousand among girls fifteen to nineteen years old in Norway in 1997 and in Iceland in 1995. This has been achieved through the expansion of reliable sex education; confidential, high-quality family planning services; and a wide selection of contraceptive methods. Age of first intercourse has remain unchanged, but contraceptive use has increased dramatically: A 1999 study showed that in 1997, 87 percent of sexually active sixteen-year-old girls in Finland had used a condom during their previous intercourse (Nordic Family Planning Associations, 1999).

Countries that have a high abortion rate, in contrast, have no sex education programs or have local programs that are narrow in scope, often as a result of the continuous struggle against the prevailing conservatism. The urgency inspired by the HIV epidemic has helped stimulate sex education but with questionable effectiveness (Eggleston et al., 2000; Population Council, 2001). This can be attributed, at least in part, to inadequate training of the personnel in charge of its implementation. In fact, resistance to sex education programs often comes from parents and teachers, who may be called upon to participate in sex education programs and who feel uncomfortable speaking in public about sexuality and reproduction.

A recent analysis of the increasing amount of information available from evaluations of sex education programs shows that their effective promotion of responsible sexual behavior can result in postponement of the initiation of sexual activity and increased use of contraceptives among adolescents who are sexually active (Irwin, 2004). This result reinforces the conclusion that by helping to reduce gender power imbalance and promote mutual respect about sexual decisions, sex education contributes to the reduction of unintended pregnancy and abortion (Nordic Family Planning Associations, 1999; Moore, 2000).

The relationship of the abortion rate to sex education, contraception, and the legal status of abortion is illustrated in Figure 11.4 (Henshaw, Singh, and Haas, 1999), which compares three groups of countries. The first group comprises three western European countries with very low abortion rates, where there is broad access to legal abortion, to sex education, and to contraception. The second group is made up of three Latin American countries with an intermediate level of abortion rates, where

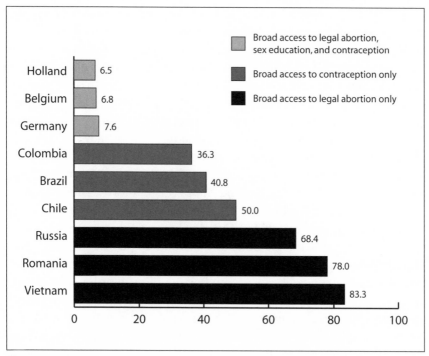

Figure 11.4. Abortion rate per thousand women of childbearing age and access to legal abortion, to broad-based sex education, and to methods of contraception. Source: Henshaw, Singh, and Haas, 1999.

there is wide access to contraceptives but where access to legal abortion is restricted and sex education is inadequate. The third group includes three countries with very high abortion rates, where there is broad access to legal abortion but where access to contraception and sex education is inadequate. Clearly, broad access to contraception and adequate sex education are required to achieve low abortion rates, while liberal or restrictive legislations appear to have no influence over the incidence of abortion.

Social Support for Motherhood

The interventions described, which aimed to reduce the number of abortions, all relate to prevention of unwanted pregnancy. Under certain circumstances, however, prevention of pregnancy is not possible. For example, an abortion may result from a pregnancy that was wanted until a negative reaction from the woman's social group made it unsustainable (Alvarez et al., 1999; Ehrenfeld, 1999).

If we look at the reasons that women give for choosing abortion, we will see that they might have continued their pregnancies if they had had more support from their families and from society in general (Ehrenfeld, 1999). It is not uncommon for young, unmarried women who become pregnant to have done so with the conscious or subconscious desire to have a child. A woman in this situation may have a permanent partner or a cherished boyfriend. She may delight in the news of her pregnancy and expect to be able to continue her education or her career, with the support of her partner and family. The couple may or may not continue their lives together, and may or may not marry, but what allows the woman to have the baby is the social, economic and emotional support of her immediate family. When that support is not forthcoming, women often see pregnancy termination as the only alternative, as in the case of young *Luisa* in the story told in Chapter 1.

Sometimes, for one or both of the woman's parents, the idea that their daughter engaged in premarital sex and that their friends and acquaintances will know is more than they can bear. In order to hide from the public what they consider to be dishonorable behavior, they may insist on either an abortion or the marriage of the expectant couple. The young woman may welcome marriage, particularly if it does not oblige her to abandon previous life plans or if she can share the responsibilities of motherhood with her mother or with another family member. Unfortunately, however, forced marriages rarely succeed in forming a long-standing family unit (McCarthy and Menken, 1979; Billy, Landale, and McLaughlin, 1986).

Support is needed not only from the family but also from society at large. The unmarried pregnant adolescent will require a receptive response from school administrators in order to continue her studies. Otherwise, she will be put in the position of having to decide either to give birth, discontinue her studies, and forsake her personal ambitions or to abort. Even older women, who may already have children and who may want another baby, may have to decide between aborting and losing a job that is incompatible with pregnancy, delivery, breastfeeding, and child care (Casas, 1996).

Society must ensure that a pregnant adolescent who wishes to have a baby does not have to interrupt her studies in order to do so and that a pregnant woman will not lose her job, will receive appropriate care during pregnancy and delivery, and will not have to make the choice either to continue her career or to breastfeed and care for her baby.

The prevention of abortion among adolescent girls is also contingent on the education of the society in which they live. Society as a whole, and parents in particular, must understand sexuality and human sexual behavior, bearing in mind the sexual activity or sexual repression of their own youths, if they are to understand the behavior of their adolescent children. Despite the difficulty of the task of cultivating a healthy attitude toward sexuality, and despite considerable resistance from some sectors, progress has been achieved in many countries (Gibbs, 1991; Amaral, 2002; Overington, 2002).

The establishment of mechanisms to help pregnant women stay in school—with sufficient flexibility to compensate for absence from class during the final weeks of pregnancy, during delivery, and during the immediate postpartum period—can clearly contribute to the prevention of abortion. The creation of systems to motivate and compensate the employers of pregnant women during pregnancy, delivery, and the postpartum period are also necessary. Legislation to improve compliance with existing laws that support pregnancy and breastfeeding and to make child care available to working mothers should also be considered.

Policymakers and opinion leaders, especially those who are zealous in their opposition to abortion, must recognize that the introduction of these social changes is essential to the reduction of the abortion rates in their communities.

12

How to Reduce the Human, Social, and Economic Costs of Abortion

It is quite obvious that the human, social, and economic costs of induced abortion would be reduced if if there were fewer abortions in the world. Even if all the proposed measures were universally implemented, however, a significant number of induced abortions would undoubtedly take place in the foreseeable future.

The actions required to reduce the negative consequences of induced abortion can be summarized in four words: *Make all abortions safe.* That is to say, if we succeed in providing every woman who is unable to avoid the decision to terminate her pregnancy with access to abortion under safe conditions and in a hospitable environment, the negative consequences of induced abortion will be dramatically reduced (Sundstrom, 1996). In order to achieve this goal, abortions must be legal, safe, and open—just another omponent of a woman's reproductive health care—and women who decide to abort must have the understanding and support of society.

A number of social and political changes are required to fulfill this objective: First, unwanted pregnancy must become the exception to the rule in women's lives; second, women who want to have a child should receive the support of society; and third, women who see no alternative to pregnancy termination should have access to safe and hospitable services. Chapter 11 considered the first two conditions. We now turn to the third.

Improving Women's Status in Society

Those who defend women's rights often argue that if men had to suffer the consequences of unsafe abortion, safe abortion would already be universally available—that is, that societies have not paid due attention to the problem because it affects only women, who in many societies are treated as second-class citizens. The illegality of abortion affects all women, regardless of their social and economic status, but women in the higher social classes have the means to secure an illegal but safe abortion, whereas women of limited means are forced to expose themselves to the risks of unsafe abortion. Therefore, women in the higher socioeconomic strata, who have greater influence and power, are less motivated to change abortion laws, whereas those who have the double disadvantage of being female and poor have little or no power to influence political decisions in their societies (Diallo et al., 2000).

The predominant indifference of men with respect to the problem is highlighted by the facility with which they can disengage themselves from any responsibility for the pregnancy. Bethania Avila, a feminist Brazilian leader, graphically synthesized this male detachment from their reproductive responsibilities: "Men abort with their mouths. They just say, 'It is not mine!' " So clear and strong was this message, that it has remained with Aníbal Faúndes for the twenty-plus years since he first heard the words spoken at the Latin American Workshop on Population and Health, Campinas, SP, Brazil, September 1985. Although paternity can now be accurately determined, only a minuscule proportion of the world's population has access to this technology.

As women gain recognition as citizens with rights equal to those of men, access to safe abortion for all women improves. The greater the power and political influence of women, the better the chance that they will not be punished for pregnancy termination. Consequently, in countries where women have gained a more egalitarian position in society, induced abortions tend to be safer. Improving women's status in society is clearly required to reduce the human, personal, and economic costs of abortion. When women's status is raised, the abortion rate will drop, the safety of the procedure will improve, and women's sexual and reproductive rights will be respected.

In recent decades, great political progress has been made toward the recognition of women's reproductive rights. The two key events were the 1994 Cairo Conference on Population and Development and the 1995 Beijing Conference on Women (United Nations, 1995a, 1995b). The Cairo Conference, rejecting demographic targets, placed great emphasis on development, education, and employment. Even more important, it gave high priority to gender equity and women's sexual and reproductive rights. Specific reference to abortion was made as follows:

In no case should [abortion] be promoted as a method of family planning. All Governments and relevant intergovernmental and non-governmental organizations are urged to strengthen their commitment to women's health, to deal with the health impact of unsafe abortion as a major public health concern and to reduce the recourse to abortion through expanded and improved family-planning services. Prevention of unwanted pregnancies must always be given the highest priority and every attempt should be made to eliminate the need for abortion. Women who have unwanted pregnancies should have ready access to reliable information and compassionate counseling. Any measures or changes related to abortion within the health system can only be determined at the national or local level according to the national legislative process. In circumstances where abortion is not against the law, such abortion should be safe. In all cases, women should have access to quality services for the management of complications arising from abortion. Post-abortion counseling, education and family-planning services should be offered promptly, which will also help to avoid repeat abortion. (United Nations, 1995a, p. 44)

The Beijing Conference ratified the Cairo agreements and went one step further, urging governments to consider reviewing laws that punish women who have undergone illegal abortions (United Nations, 1995b). The Cairo and Beijing agreements set clear guidelines about the measures necessary to position women as citizens with rights equal to those of men. Implementation of the agreements, however, has lagged far behind expectations.

Decriminalizing or Extending Legal Grounds for Abortion

The most rational, effective way to reduce the human, social, and economic costs of abortion is to abolish the laws and codes that penalize the voluntary termination of pregnancy. At the same time, however—as the experience of eastern Europe, Vietnam, and Cuba has shown—all methods for the prevention of unwanted pregnancy must be made available and accessible.

As we have seen, whereas virtually all legal abortions are safe, the vast majority of illegal abortions are unsafe. The negative consequences of the criminalization of abortion were dramatically illustrated by the increase in maternal mortality after Romania's November 1965 prohibition of both abortion and contraceptives (see Chapter 4). Even more dramatic was the effect of the decriminalization of abortion and contraception after the fall of Nicolae Ceaucescu in December 1989: Abortion-related maternal mortality fell from about 150 per 100,000 live births in the previous year to fewer than 50 per 100,000 live births two years after decriminalization (Stephenson et al., 1992; WHO, 1997) (Figure 12.1). Th Romanian experience best illustrates the positive effect that the restoration of induced abortion and contraception as legal medical procedures has on abortion-related maternal mortality.

Th e relative safety of legal abortion and the severe consequences c backdoor abortion have been documented in several other countries as well. In England and Wales, for example, there were no deaths related to induced abortion between 1982 and 1984—following passage of the Abortion Act, which extended the legal grounds for abortion and greatly facilitated free access to safe abortion—compared with 75 to 80 deaths per triennium before the act was passed (Stephenson et al., 1992). Th same trend occurred in the state of New York. In the two years after the 1970 liberalization of abortion laws, there was a 50 percent drop in the number of abortion-related maternal deaths (Tietze, Pakter, and Berger,

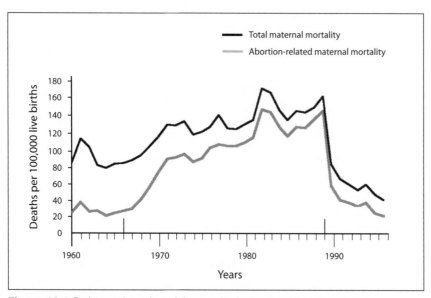

Figure 12.1. Total maternal mortality and abortion-related maternal mortality in Romania during years abortion was legal (pre-1966), the years during which abortion was illegal (1966–1989), and when it was again legal (post-1989). Source: Stephenson et al., 1992; WHO, 1997.

1973). Data from the United States confirm the dramatic decrease in abortion-related maternal mortality following the Supreme Court's 1973 *Roe v. Wade* decision (Cates, Grimes, and Schulz, 2003).

Improving Access to Legal Abortion

As we saw in Chapter 4, the decriminalization of abortion does not guarantee easy access to safe procedures. Without diminishing the importance of advocating for more liberal laws, and although such liberalization has occurred, we strongly believe that too little emphasis has been placed on the implementation of existing laws. Bonnie Campbell, the director of the Violence against Women Office of the U.S. Justice Department, has commented with respect to domestic violence laws, "It does not matter how good the law is unless you can change the attitude of the people enforcing the law" (quoted in Gleick and County, 1996, p. 13).

In the case of laws related to abortion, the "people enforcing the laws" are mostly public health officials and gynecologists/obstetricians. The lack of respect for existing laws in many countries indicates that those responsible for the public health system have not made it a priority to mitigate the human drama of abortion. It also indicates a lack of sensitivity on the part of gynecologists/obstetricians to the suffering and to the needs of women who meet the conditions required by law and who desperately want to terminate their pregnancies (Faúndes and Torres, 2002).

In some countries where laws have been liberalized, for example— such as India, Zambia, and (to a lesser degree) South Africa—the majority of women still do not have access to safe abortion services. In these countries, it is essential to accelerate the process of adapting and upgrading the public health system to meet the demand for voluntary pregnancy terminations. It is important to reiterate, however, that access to safe abortion services must be accompanied by efforts to reduce the number of unwanted pregnancies.

Limited access to abortion services is not a problem singularly distinctive of developing countries with minimal resources. Despite the liberal legal status of abortion guaranteed by the U.S. Supreme Court, for example, low-income women in the United States cannot easily access legal abortion. A lack of public resources for the provision of abortion services makes access painfully limited for many U.S. women. At the same time, the fact that the pregnancy rate among adolescents is several times higher in the United States than in western Europe can be explained, at least in part, by the limited access to and even legal restriction against contraceptive information and services in public facilities for this age group.

Although access to contraception is important for the population as a whole, certain groups, such as women who request pregnancy termination, require special treatment. Epidemiological studies from decades past showed that the chance of having an induced abortion is much higher among women who have done so in the past (Requena, 1966). Consequently, the care of women who use safe abortion services is not complete without appropriate contraceptive and sex education and immediate provision of a full range of methods of birth control. Adolescents require special treatment because—honestly convinced that they will never be in the same position again—they frequently reject post-abortion contraception. Unfortunately, studies show that repeat abortion is more frequent among young adolescent women even when they have received post-abortion counseling and services (Hardy and Herud, 1975).

Where abortion is permitted only under limited circumstances, women who fulfill the legal requirements may not have access to safe pregnancy termination. In these regions, access to safe abortion greatly depends on how liberally or restrictively the law is interpreted by society. A crucial role is played by obstetricians/gynecologists, since ultimately it is they who decide whether or not to perform the abortion, and by the legal profession, whose function it is to interpret the law.

Improving access to safe abortion to the full extent permitted by law is an important mechanism for reducing the consequences of induced abortion. Brazil provides an example of a successful effort to improve access to legal abortion within the parameters of restrictive laws. Current legislation allows physicians to perform abortions under two conditions: (1) if the pregnancy resulted from a rape or (2) if the pregnancy seriously endangers the woman's life.

Since the early 1980s, women's organizations and a handful of gynecologists/obstetricians in Brazil had been raising awareness about the need to provide care for women who requested legal abortions. In 1987 and 1988, the cities of Rio de Janeiro and São Paulo established specific services for the care of women who requested legal abortion. Although the services were not effectively implemented in Rio, they worked reasonably well in São Paulo (Colás et al., 1994). In addition, a university hospital in the city of Campinas began providing these services in the early 1980s. Until 1995, these were the only public services available for

Brazil's population of 170 million. The number of women victims of rape who obtained a legal abortion was extremely small, no more than twenty to thirty per year.

Since 1996, under the initiative of one of the authors (AF), Cemicamp (a nongovernmental organization working in reproductive health and rights) had joined forces with women's groups and with the Brazilian Federation of Obstetrical and Gynecological Societies (FEBRASGO) to promote the provision of legal abortion services in public hospitals. An important immediate result was FEBRASGO's 1997 creation of the National Scientific Commission on Sexual Violence and Abortion According to the Law. FEBRASGO's official seal of approval on the initiative was highly significant for Brazilian gynecologists/obstetricians. Cemicamp and the FEBRASGO committee worked together to motivate gynecologists/obstetricians and health authorities to establish clear procedures for implementing the existing abortion law, particularly for women victims of rape. In 1998 the Ministry of Health officially sanctioned these procedures, and from 1999 it has joined forces with Cemicamp, FEBRASGO, and the women's rights movement in an effort to provide access to legal abortion (Faúndes, Leocádio, and Andalaft-Neto, 2002). From 1996 to the end of 2002, the number of public hospitals that provide specialized care to women who experience sexual violence increased from four to more than two hundred. Because many of these are teaching hospitals, the culture has already begun to change for future physicians. In addition, the topic of gender violence and legal abortion has become a constant fixture at scientific meetings on obstetrics and gynecology in the country. The key to this spectacular success was the alliance of the medical establishment, the women's rights movement, and the federal government.

During the process it became clear that the support of peers is essential to the comfort of health professionals in providing abortion services and that health professionals can count on the support of their peers once they understand that the goal is not to promote abortion but to prevent women from running the risk of complications and death from unsafe procedures.

A Fairer, More Liberal Interpretation of the Law

Whereas in many countries women who fulfill the legal requirements do not have access to safe abortions, in other countries the liberal interpretation of restrictive laws facilitates access to safe abortion. Facilitating access to safe abortion, even when the legal conditions are unclear, not only saves women's lives and prevents human suffering but also conserves valuable and often scarce health resources (Konje, Obisesan, and Ladipo, 1992).

In Mozambique, for example, the law is quite restrictive, but the health system's interpretation of the law allows access to safe abortions for women who would otherwise have to resort to unsafe methods. One of the authors (AF) witnessed the process that led to this courageous and compassionate initiative:

> I visited Mozambique for the first time in 1980, just two years after it gained independence from Portugal. Because the Portuguese had, until 1978, occupied all positions for which any level of education was required, the country was left with virtually no professionally or technically skilled personnel following independence. There were just over a hundred physicians, most of them foreigners, in a country of about twelve million inhabitants. There was one medical school and not enough candidates who had completed secondary school to fill it. As an experienced obstetrician, I spent some time (I wish it could have been more) working at the Maputo Maternity Hospital. There, to my great surprise, I met the minister of health himself, Dr. Pascoal Mocumbi, who was the obstetrician on duty. One of the few obstetricians in the country, he had declined to use his government post to escape his duty to the people in need. During the day he acted as minister of health, and several nights each week, as well as some Sundays and holidays, he worked as an obstetrician at the very busy Maputo Maternity Hospital. Although to him it seemed natural, I have never seen anyone in his governmental position acting this way and I doubt whether there have been similar examples in any other countries.
>
> Combining his position as a politician with his close contact with the people as a physician gave him a unique perspective. Following its Portuguese heritage, Mozambique had adopted restrictive abortion laws. As a result, Dr. Mocumbi had to provide care to women who suffered serious complications from backdoor abortions. He witnessed, in large numbers, the suffering and often the death of the women who came to the hospital every day with severe bleeding or infections. In fact abortion-related death occurred almost every week. As minister of health, his reaction was to promote, plan, and implement (with the limited human resources available) an

extensive and well-organized family planning program, specifically
aimed at reducing maternal mortality and abortion. It was clear to
Dr. Mocumbi that criminalization of abortion was responsible for a
good part of the suffering he witnessed, but he knew that to change
the law would be a long process that would consume time and energy
better used to accomplish other urgent tasks. Thus, courageously
taking it upon himself to interpret the law, he dictated a ministerial
order authorizing public hospitals to practice abortion when
pregnancy put the woman's life at risk and when it was the result of
contraceptive failure. This meant, in practice, a broad acceptance of
pregnancy termination. The obstetrician in charge of the Maputo
Maternity Hospital, well aware of the problem, put the minister
of health's instructions into practice at once. As word of this new
service spread, it was requested by an increasing number of women.
Consequently, within a year, the number of women dying from
abortion complications was drastically reduced.

This is a wonderful example of the difference between adopting policies based on firsthand experience with a social and health problem and
discussing an issue behind the closed doors of a government cabinet,
far from the harsh realities of the people. When a leader in a position of
power has direct contact with the dramatic consequences of the criminalization of abortion, his or her political position on the issue takes on
a totally different character.

The number of safe abortions performed at the Maputo Maternity
Hospital now exceeds, by far, the number of women with complications
from unsafe abortions, at a much lower cost in human suffering and
health service resources (Bugalho, 1995). Dr. Mocumbi's liberal interpretation of the law was restricted to Maputo Maternity Hospital for about
two decades, but in recent years its clear role in decreasing human suffering and saving lives and resources has led to its progressive expansion
to other cities and towns.

In the early 1970s, one of the authors (AF) was involved in a similar
process in a large public hospital in Santiago, Chile:

At the time, Chile had a very well structured public National Health
Service that provided care to 85 percent of the country's population.
The Barros Luco Hospital provided in-hospital care to the southern
districts of Santiago, serving a population of low socioeconomic
status and high fertility. In 1959, as a result of the spontaneous

response of a group of physicians and midwives to the demand of the population, this hospital had become a pioneer in introducing contraception to Chile. The idea was to prevent unwanted and high-risk pregnancies and, consequently, induced abortion and other obstetrical complications. At the time, neither the U.S. government, with its development assistance, nor the United Nations was interested in fertility regulation.

An educational program on the risks of abortion and the methods for its prevention was started in 1965 and expanded in subsequent years. The number of women with abortion complications admitted to the Barros Luco Hospital was reduced from more than five thousand a year to slightly more than thirty-two hundred in 1972. Nevertheless, fifteen women died from septic post-abortion complications; many young, childless women lost their uterus, ovaries, and fallopian tubes, leaving them sterile; and, in spite of educational efforts to encourage the use of contraception, multiple cases of repeat abortions continued to be identified.

At this point, the public had become better informed about abortion, and its social significance was changing. At the same time, the government had pointed out that the struggle against induced abortion had to consider the "eventual legalization of abortion . . . and more immediately . . . an expansion of the criteria for therapeutic abortion, as in the cases of contraceptive failure" (Allende, 1971).

In 1971, the change in public attitude toward abortion and the high incidence of unwanted pregnancies resulting from contraceptive failure led a group of physicians working at the Barros Luco Hospital to make a bold decision: They started to perform free therapeutic abortions for patients referred by contraceptive clinics within the hospital's catchment area whose pregnancies were the result of contraceptive failure. The justification for the legality as "therapeutic abortion" was that it was documented in the patient's record that the pregnancy was unwanted, had occurred during use of a contraceptive, and that the patient would inevitably have an induced abortion. The logical medical procedure was to perform a safe abortion rather than expose the woman to the risks of a pregnancy termination at the hands of an unskilled abortionist.

A committee was assigned the task of evaluating each application for "therapeutic" pregnancy termination. In order to comply with the Chilean law that allowed therapeutic abortion when pregnancy seriously imperiled the patient's health or life, the reasons for the abortions were documented and signed by at least two physicians (Isaacs and Sanhueza, 1975).

The situation continued unchanged for several months, but then, as the committee became increasingly strict, a series of dramatic events occurred: After their initial applications were rejected, a young woman committed suicide, and a nurse's aide from the hospital was admitted with serious post-abortion sepsis. As a result of these and several other similar, though less dramatic cases, the rules were changed. The decision to accept or reject an application to terminate a pregnancy became the responsibility of the Abortion Section. The only conditions were the following: Gestation could not be over twelve weeks, the applicants were required to prove that they lived within the hospital's catchment area, and the women had to agree to use an effective post-abortion contraceptive.

The workload in the abortion clinic increased exponentially, from eighty-nine abortion-related operations to nearly five hundred in six months. This short time also saw a marked change in the profile of the usual client. Women of higher economic status now requested pregnancy termination as well. In addition, since it was not difficult to obtain a certificate that "proved" that a patient lived within the catchment area, women from all over Santiago and women from the countryside put in their requests. Naturally, this increase in the number of operations meant a great increase in the workload for the entire staff, but they accepted their lot because they understood that they were fulfilling a mission that went far beyond their usual duties.

From January through August 1973, there was only one maternal death due to post-induced abortion complications in the Barros Luco Hospital maternity ward—a patient who had had an induced abortion in another area. During the same period in 1972, nine women had died from abortion-related complications.

Meanwhile, media reports continued to reflect the changes that were taking place in Chilean society. In March and September 1973, a widely read, influential women's magazine, Paula, published a series of interviews with women from different social backgrounds and with physicians who were also university professors, explaining why they were in favor of legalizing abortion. Two of the most widely circulated newspapers in Santiago, *La Tercera de la Hora* and *La Segunda*, published full-page articles reporting that pregnancies were being terminated in a hospital in Santiago to prevent unsafe abortions and their many negative consequences. Surprisingly, despite the general belief at the time that public opinion morally opposed pregnancy termination under any circumstances, virtually no negative reaction from the public was forthcoming.

The Barros Luco Hospital's liberal interpretation of the existing law came to an abrupt end with the 1973 military coup (Faúndes and Hardy, 1978). Within a few years, the government had changed the constitution, and Chile became one of the two countries in Latin America where abortion is completely prohibited by law. It does not, however, prevent Chile from having one of the highest abortion rates in the region (Singh and Wulf, 1994).

Several other countries currently interpret their abortion laws in ways that allow broad access to safe abortion. In Bangladesh, with its very restrictive abortion law, "menstrual regulation" is permitted, within the limits of the country's capacity, with virtually no exception (Kabir, 1989; Begum, 1993).

Access to High Quality Post-Abortion Care

As long as abortion remains a crime and access to safe, compassionate abortion services is not readily available, unsafe, backdoor abortions will continue to occur in large numbers. Because this situation is, unfortunately, likely to remain unchanged in many countries for some time, it is important to look to post-abortion care as a way to reduce the human costs of unsafe abortion (WHO, 1995; Winkler, Oliveras, and McIntosh, 1995). As we saw in Chapter 4, when an abortion is performed under inadequate technical and hygienic conditions, heavy bleeding, infection, or both frequently result. Hospitals that fail to provide safe abortion services must then care for women who suffer the complications that result from backdoor abortions and do everything within their power to save the women's lives. The difference between life and death for a woman with complications depends on her ability to access quality care. Most deaths result from delay in seeking treatment and from the incapacity or unwillingness of health systems to provide life-saving services.

Access to hospitals for women who suffer from abortion complications is not always readily available. In Bolivia, a qualitative assessment coordinated by the Ministry of Health in collaboration with WHO, found that access to services for post-abortion care could be limited. According to the researchers, in some hospitals, particularly those run by the Catholic Church, women suspected of having had an induced abortion were turned away (Camacho et al., 1996). Discrimination against and mistreatment of women who sought post-abortion care have also been observed by human rights groups in Argentina (Chiarotti et al, 2003).

Recently, Dora Byamukama, a parliamentarian and chairperson of Law Uganda, addressed a workshop on women's rights and the law, commenting, "Many girls and women have died of abortion related problems due to fear of going to hospitals and being denounced to the police" (quoted in Nankinga, 2002). At least in some countries, women had good reason to be fearful. According to the Chilean Ministry of Justice, between 1980 and 1989, 1,939 people were prosecuted for having participated in some way in an induced abortion (Casas, 1996). Women were denounced by personnel at the hospital where they received post-abortion care, usually at the personal initiative of just one pro-life person, and many of them were jailed. Thus, access to post-abortion care can be limited by providers in two ways: by direct rejection or by the threat that women who have had an induced abortion may be prosecuted.

Even if care is provided to women with abortion complications, the quality of this care can pale compared to the quality of care provided for other reasons. A study in Mexico that evaluated the quality of care for women with abortion complications found that only 17 percent knew which physician performed the curettage or vacuum aspiration and less than 5 percent were informed about the use of post-abortion medication or possible complications following discharge (Langer et al., 1999).

Most countries agree that women who have undergone an abortion need emergency care and that this care must be provided even when there are legal restrictions to induced abortion. In the words of the Cairo Conference, "In all cases women should have access to quality services for the management of complications arising from abortion" (United Nations, 1995a, p. 44). Assessment of the woman's condition and provision of services should be available on a twenty-four-hour basis and should be provided with the urgency required by the severity of the condition (WHO, 1995).

It is beyond the purview of this book to discuss the technical aspects of emergency care for women who suffer complications following induced abortions; these have been described in detail in various technical publications (WHO, 1995; Winkler, Oliveras, and McIntosh, 1995). Our purpose is to highlight the fact that the prevalent discrimination against women who have induced abortions has led to inadequate emergency care and that this neglect adds to the human, social, and economic costs of unsafe abortion (Nankinga, 2002).

A More Positive Attitude Among
Health Care Workers

The authors have witnessed in emergency care facilities the inhumane and cruel treatment of women suspected of induced abortion, as has been reported in many publications (Casas, 1996; Maforah, Wood, and Jewkes, 1997). This kind of treatment is tied to the moral condemnation of women who have induced abortions that takes place in many societies, particularly in those countries where high fertility ideals still prevail or where lower fertility ideals have only recently begun to take hold (Billings et al., 1999). Although it is difficult to generalize, and some improvement has been noted in various countries, the negative attitude lingers, particularly where restrictive abortion laws exist (Casas, 1996).

Some studies have reported successful efforts to overcome the negative mindset of providers through training (Langer et al., 1999). It appears that the attitude of providers is strongly influenced by the criminalization of induced abortion. The perception is that if induced abortion is considered a crime under existing law, most of society must oppose induced abortion. The laws that condemn women also imply that those who have had induced abortions have chosen to do so out of selfishness and cruelty, and despite the availability of other alternatives. Thus, it is easy for providers to adopt the position of defenders of the fetus and the persecutors of the women who dare to reject their potential children (Maforah, Wood, and Jewkes, 1997; Billings et al., 1999).

Although a positive change in the provider's attitude can be achieved through training, only a change in the attitude of society as a whole will bring any real understanding. A hospitable environment in the emergency services will reduce both the physical and emotional costs to women who undergo induced abortions.

13
The Paradox
Rejecting Abortion and Opposing the
Prevention of Unwanted Pregnancies

As we have seen throughout this book, the most efficient way to prevent abortion is to avoid unwanted pregnancies. We might expect, therefore, that those who oppose abortion would be in favor of measures that are aimed at reducing unwanted pregnancy: the large-scale dissemination of complete unbiased information about all contraceptive methods and easy access to all of them; reliable contraceptive services; broad-based, unbiased sexual health education programs; and the promotion of gender power balance in relationships. Unfortunately, what we usually see is the reverse. Some of the most vocal opponents of abortion also oppose efforts to improve the availability and accessibility of modern contraceptive methods, sex education programs in schools, and the advancement of women's socioeconomic role in society (Boonstra, 2002a; Broder, 2002).

Despite the demonstrated efficacy of contraception in reducing unwanted pregnancy and abortion, for example, the current Vatican leadership and other staunchly conservative religious groups oppose the use of any modern contraceptive method. The official position of the Catholic Church is to condone only "natural" methods of fertility regulation: periodic abstinence and lactational amenorrhea (LAM).*

What is worse, groups that defend the criminalization of abortion in the name of religion do not limit their argument to moral condemnation or direct their argument toward only members of the same faith. Instead,

---

*Periodic abstinence consists of avoiding coitus at the period of the menstrual cycle during which the chances of pregnancy are greater (during the six days preceding ovulation and during the day of ovulation itself). LAM is the practice of exclusive breastfeeding during the first six months after birth (provided that menstruation does not resume within that period), which has a blocking effect on ovulation (an effect that disappears at or shortly before the first postpartum menstrual period).

they use their political influence to block access to accurate information about modern contraceptives, challenging approval of their commercialization, their continuous availability through the public health system, and the use of public funds to provide contraceptives for low-income people.

Frequently, instead of acknowledging the religious basis of their opposition, they claim legal or health reasons. In countries where abortion is legally restricted, these groups have been known to make the false claim that some methods, such as the IUD and the emergency contraceptive pill, are legally unacceptable because they act by inducing an early abortion every month. To oppose the use of condoms, they have negated their proven effectiveness in preventing the transmission of sexually transmitted diseases, including AIDS (Amaral, 2002).

Opposition to "Artificial" Contraceptive Methods

As we have noted, some Christian churches, in particular the Roman Catholic Church, have condemned the use of any method that is not defined as "natural," using arguments that are based on wrong information or a distorted interpretation of scientific evidence. After the introduction of the combined oral contraceptive pill in the early 1960s, the Catholic Church spent several years internally debating its position on the subject with the possibility of approving this new contraceptive method. By the time the leadership decided to officially condemn its use, the pill had already been marketed and was being used by women all over the world, including a large number of Catholic women. This, in our view, explains why there has not been the same organized religious opposition to its use as there has been with newer contraceptive methods. Still, the opposition by the Catholic Church prevents the pill from being distributed within the large network of U.S. Catholic hospitals.

The condom, a contraceptive method that was available much earlier, was not viewed as a major problem because of its low level of use in predominantly Christian countries. With the exponential increase in the demand for condoms since the spread of HIV/AIDS, however, condom use has become a matter of concern to some Christian authorities. The argument to oppose its use is the claim that condoms are ineffective in the prevention of HIV transmission, although they are, in fact, highly effective, dramatically reducing the number of new infections in some countries (Weller and Davis, 2002; Holmes, Levine and Weaver, 2004)

Christian groups have also effectively limited access to female and male surgical sterilization, either by lobbying against liberalizing laws or by using other means of preventing their use. For example, many Catholic hospitals, which care for mostly non-Catholic populations in the United States, refuse to provide emergency contraception or perform tubal ligations or vasectomies (Catholics for a Free Choice, 2002; Gold, 2002). In areas where Catholic hospitals are the only facilities that provide surgical services, this policy effectively limits access to sterilization.

Opposition to contraceptive methods based on religious principles, a function of the right to religious freedom, merits full respect. But the corollary of religious freedom is that no religion can impose its views on those who do not profess its faith (Park Ridge Center, 1994). Moreover, there is no justification for manipulating scientific evidence to support a religious argument.

Opposition to Contraceptive Methods under the Allegation That They Induce Abortions

The argument that some contraceptive methods cause frequent and periodic abortions is based on two assumptions: (1) that pregnancy begins with fertilization of the ovum and (2) that some methods prevent pregnancy after fertilization. The question of when pregnancy begins was discussed in Chapter 2 and we accepted the biomedical definition that it starts with implantation. Moreover, this question is irrelevant if the method of contraception acts by preventing fertilization. In particular, the presumption of post-fertilization effect has been linked to the copper IUD and the emergency contraceptive pill. Current scientific evidence overwhelmingly opposes this notion, however (Croxatto et al., 2001; Croxatto, 2002b; Diaz and Croxatto, 2003). The only scientifically proven mechanisms of contraceptive action for these two methods are pre-fertilization.

As we have seen, failure of implantation of the fertilized ovum, or *zygote,* frequently occurs in nature without any outside interference. It is possible, although there is no solid scientific evidence to support the theory, that this natural event may occur somewhat more frequently with the use of some contraceptives. Even so, however, since other well-documented mechanisms of action are sufficient to explain the efficacy of these contraceptive methods, the possibility would apply to only a small number of cases.

The possibility of post-fertilization action has been raised with respect to intrauterine devices, modern hormonal methods, and even "natural" methods of fertility control—such as LAM and periodic abstinence—approved by the Catholic Church. In the case of LAM, we know that ovulation often occurs in the month preceding the return of menstruation. Women who use this method rarely become pregnant because the production of progesterone during the second half of the first ovulation after delivery is below the limits found in normal cycles (Lewis et al., 1991; Kennedy and Visness, 1992). As a result, the inner layer of the uterus—the endometrium—is not prepared to receive the zygote. There is, therefore, good reason to believe that during the month prior to the first menstruation after delivery, LAM may prevent implantation.

Similarly, it has been proposed that when a couple has sexual intercourse close to the limits of ovum viability—for example, while practicing periodic abstinence—fertilization may occur; however, the resulting zygote may not be normal due to the aging of the ovum, and it might not be implanted in the uterine wall (Wilcox, Weinberg, and Baird, 1998).

It is not our intention to claim that prevention of implantation is the main mechanism of action of these "natural" methods of family planning. This mechanism is, in fact, irrelevant compared with the inhibition of ovulation resulting from full lactation with the LAM method and the absence of sex during the fertile period with periodic abstinence. Similarly, it can be said that interference with implantation, if it occurs, is irrelevant in the case of copper IUDs. The copper ions liberated from these IUDs reach high concentrations in the cervical mucus, the uterus, and the fallopian tubes. These concentrations of copper are sufficient to immobilize and kill the spermatozoa and the ovum, preventing fertilization (Jecht and Bernstein, 1973; Tatum, 1973; Larsson and Hamberger, 1977; Koch and Vogel, 1979; Ros et al., 1979; Battersby, Chandler, and Morton, 1982). This is undoubtedly the main mechanism of action of copper bearing IUDs.

The erroneous concept that IUDs act after fertilization derives from earlier studies carried out on rodents. The placement of inert pieces of material or a copper wire in the uterus of these animals did not prevent fertilization but blocked the implantation of the fertilized eggs (Zipper, Medel, and Prager, 1969). It is easy to recover normal fertilized ova from the uterus of rodents bearing a copper wire (Zipper, Delgado, and Guiloff, 1963; Zipper, Medel, and Prager, 1969). However, studies that recovered ova from the genital tract of women following sexual intercourse at the time of ovulation were successful in obtaining fertilized ova in about half the subjects who were not using contraceptives, and the same studies failed to recover any normally fertilized ova from women who were using copper IUDs (Alvarez et al., 1988; Ortiz, Croxatto, and Bardin, 1996). These results give further support to the notion that prevention of implantation is not relevant in humans and that the contraceptive effect of the copper IUD is mediated by the deleterious activity of copper over both gametes (sperm and ovum) (Ortiz, Croxatto, and Bardin, 1996; Araya et al., 2003).

The same can be said of emergency contraception (EC). The initial hypothesis was that the contraceptive steroids used in EC would alter the characteristics of the endometrium in such a way that implantation would be blocked, but this hypothesis has not been confirmed. Samples of the endometrium from women who had taken the EC pill were collected at the expected time of implantation. The histological study of the samples, using electron microscopy and histochemistry, failed to identify any alteration that might interfere with implantation (Durand et al., 2001; Marions et al., 2002). This was not surprising, considering that the progestagens used in the EC pills received their names because they produce endometrial changes similar to those caused by progesterone in the normal cycle, which are needed for implantation and continuation of pregnancy. Moreover, these synthetic hormones are called "pro-ge-stagens" because of their ability to maintain pregnancy in animals that have had their ovaries removed after implantation.

Recent studies (Croxatto et al., 2004) have shown that by suppressing the surge of luteinizing hormone the pituitary hormone that triggers ovulation, the EC pills inhibit ovulation for at least five days, which is the maximum period of sperm survival in the woman's body. This effect is not observed if the EC is administered within the forty-eight hours prior to ovulation. In that case, however, EC has the additional effect of interfering with the ovum's capacity to be fertilized. Finally, progestagens have a proven inhibitory effect on the sperm's ability to migrate and to fertilize the ovum (Nikkanen et al., 2000; Croxatto, 2002b).

These proven pre-fertilization effects of the EC pills are sufficient to explain their contraceptive effectiveness. Furthermore, implantation occurs between eight and twelve days after sexual intercourse, and the progestagens in the EC pills reach their highest blood level twenty-four to thirty-six hours after administration, virtually disappearing three to four days later (Johansson et al., 2002). If the action of the EC pill were inhibition of implantation, the pill would be more effective if used between six and ten days after sexual intercourse. The fact that the EC's effectiveness approaches 100 percent only when the pill is taken within twenty-four hours after sex and becomes virtually ineffective five days later strongly opposes the theory that EC acts through prevention of implantation (WHO, 1998; Croxatto, 2002b; von Hertzen et al., 2002). More recently, studies done with *Cebus apella* monkeys showed that, as in humans, EC blocked ovulation but could not avoid pregnancy if administered after fertilization (Ortiz et al., 2004)

Unfortunately, when the mechanisms of action for the IUD and the EC pill were unknown, early textbooks on contraception proposed interference with implantation as the principal mechanism of action for both. Once this hypothesis was published in authoritative texts, it was considered definitive fact and continued to be cited from one textbook to the next without critical revision based on new evidence.

In their efforts to prevent the commercialization and use of modern contraceptive methods, those who, as a matter of principle, oppose all but the "natural" methods of contraception have disregarded this new evidence and adhered to outdated information. With arguments based on wrong information, they have influenced national and local political leaders and have successfully blocked general public access to these important contraceptive methods (Harris, 2004). Through these ethically questionable means, they have influenced the behavior of women and men who do not share their values and have unwittingly contributed to the number of unwanted pregnancies and abortions.

Opposition to Sex Education

The efforts by some pro-life groups to oppose abortion prevention have not been limited to anti-contraception activities. They have opposed virtually every social change that is needed to prevent unwanted pregnancy as well. Under the misguided impression that knowledge about sexual health stimulates premature sexual activity, for example, they have opposed the implementation of broad-based, unbiased sex education programs in schools (Gibbs, 1991). They also oppose women's participation in social and economic activities, arguing that it will contribute to the disruption of the family unit and that the main role of women is to have babies and take care of their husband, children and the home in general.

The argument that sexual health education in schools and access to contraception for teenagers stimulates earlier initiation of and more frequent sexual activity (Sathe, 1994) has not been confirmed by published studies (Kirby, 2001; Kirby et al., 1993). On the other hand, the effectiveness of sex education and access to contraception in preventing pregnancy among adolescents has been repeatedly confirmed (Bromham and Oloto, 1997; Grunseit, 1997; Nordic Family Planning Associations, 1999; Kirby, 2001).

Moreover, according to some studies, appropriate sex education is associated with the postponement, rather than the anticipation, of the initiation of sexual activity and with a decrease in the number of sexually active adolescents (Mbizvo et al., 1997; Middleman, 1999). This should come as no surprise: The successful promotion of responsibility and mutual respect among adolescents of both sexes should be expected to diminish the imposition of sexual acts by adolescent boys on unwilling or uncertain adolescent girls (Underwood et al., 2001).

Opposition to comprehensive sex education has been particularly strong in the United States, whereas western European countries have a long tradition of open-minded, broad-based sex education programs that are begun early in life. An international comparison indicating that the pregnancy rate among adolescents was two to five times lower in western European countries than in the United States (Singh and Darroch, 2000) suggests the benefits of the western Europe policies in abortion reduction. A recent publication puts forth solid criticism of the official U.S. policy with respect to sex education (Stewart, Shields, and Hwang, 2004)

Abortion-Promoting Effects of "Anti-abortion" Politics

The political influence of anti-abortion groups can have disastrous effects by increasing dramatically the number of unwanted pregnancies and abortions. The decision of the George W. Bush administration to withhold the annual $34 million U.S. contribution to the UN Population Fund (UNFPA) is estimated will result in about two million unwanted pregnancies, eight hundred thousand more abortions, and forty-seven hundred more maternal deaths per year. The basis for the decision was the assumption that UNFPA was condoning or even supporting forced abortions in China, an assumption that was challenged by the report of a three-person team sent to China by the Bush administration itself. According to the report, they did not "find any evidence that UNFPA had knowingly supported or participated in the management of a program of coercive abortion or involuntary sterilization in the People's Republic of China" (quoted in Broder, 2002, p. D-3) This report confirmed the findings of another group that had previously been sent to China by the

United Kingdom for the same purpose. Nevertheless, the assessments were not enough to appease the "anti-abortion" movement. Ironically and paradoxically, no other organization has done more than UNFPA to replace abortion with family planning in China. As a result, those who call themselves opponents of abortion have, instead, helped to increase the number of abortions in China and in the rest of the developing world.

Through their successful political pressure in support of the "abstinence only" sex education policy, the same groups have also contributed to the U.S. rate of adolescent pregnancy and abortion—the highest rate in the developed world (Singh and Darroch, 2000). There is general agreement on the benefits of promoting abstinence, but the dissemination of information on the prevention of pregnancy and disease for those who are sexually active is also essential, as is the understanding that sexuality is a fundamental quality of human life, important for health, happiness, individual development, and the preservation of the human race.

The universal reality is that some adolescents will remain abstinent and others will become sexually active. A policy that withholds information on protection against pregnancy and disease will only contribute to maintaining high rates of unwanted pregnancy and abortion among U.S. adolescents. More than one hundred organizations, including many of the most prestigious medical and educational associations in the United States, have called for sex education programs that include both promotion of abstinence and increased awareness of methods of protection against sexually transmitted disease and unintended pregnancy (Boonstra, 2002b). This position is founded on a broad-based review of the existing literature showing the effectiveness of these programs in reducing abortion. Meanwhile, by using their political strength to ensure the exclusion of information about contraception from U.S. sex education programs, anti-abortion groups have contributed to thousands of abortions every year.

We have great hope that a better understanding of the issues will soon become a reality for opponents of abortion, particularly those within the Catholic Church. There are so many theologians, bishops and priests who are well aware of this paradox that, sooner or later they will succeed in making the Vatican understand that the policy of opposing contraception only serves to increase the number of abortions.

PART IV
Seeking a Consensus

14

How to Reach a Consensus on Abortion

In 1997, I (AF) had the opportunity to organize a meeting on abortion for Latin American gynecologists and obstetricians, which included parliamentarians, jurists, ethicists, and women's rights advocates as well. About forty people sat around the table for two days, discussing the social problem of abortion and proposing possible solutions. An objective account of the abortion situation in the region was presented and possible actions that could help improve the situation were discussed. Well into the second day of the meeting, a female parliamentarian from Chile raised her hand to ask for the floor. Her contribution—short and to the point—remains engraved in my memory:

"I believe this meeting is of the utmost importance, and I am fully sympathetic to the problem of women who undergo induced abortions. I feel, however, that something is missing from this discussion and you should understand that I come from Chile. For two days now, all I have heard is talk of women's rights and the consequences of abortion for women. This is quite the opposite of what I have been hearing in the Chilean Parliament over the past few years. There only the fetus exists, and all discussions center on the fetus's right to life. I wonder whether these discussions would not be more constructive if at this meeting we take care not to forget the fetus and in my parliament we do not forget the woman."

This statement was among the most important of the entire meeting. It was a very clear invitation to accept diversity of values and to recognize that progress in dialogue cannot be achieved if some of the actors ignore the arguments of others, instead of making an integral analysis of the problem.

The Social Need for an "Overlapping Consensus"

Throughout history all societies have experimented with different forms of organization, with the general aim of promoting peace among their members and improving their well-being. Different forms of organization have been inspired by a variety of ideologies and value systems, usually modulated by the cultural and religious traditions of each particular society. Many models have been adopted, but none has been universally accepted.

The evolution of the organization of human societies shows a historical tendency toward increased recognition of the need to respect individual rights and to promote social justice. Perhaps the greatest difficulty in organizing a just society has been to satisfy, in an equitable manner, the aspirations of individuals with those of society—in other words, to achieve the right balance between individual good and common good or between the claims of liberty and justice.

This challenge has become progressively more urgent in recent decades as a number of circumstances have caused the world to "shrink." Technological progress, the massive and global development of communications, the increasing number of people who travel and migrate, and the globalization of the economy are forcing face-to-face interaction among people from very different cultures. Different ideologies, religions, cultures, and moral systems have to explain their differences in a rational and respectful way, both to themselves and to "the others." Inevitably, this long and difficult dialogue has tended toward identifying common values and influencing the permanent process of change that characterizes all cultures. In the process, the need to respect diversity and to develop a certain social consensus has emerged as a prerequisite to organizing a peaceful and already de facto global society.

In his last book, the late John Rawls (2001) addresses the general public, proposing "justice as fairness" as the basis for a modern democratic political system: "as a political conception of justice rather than as part of a comprehensive moral doctrine" (Rawls 2001, p. xvi). Restating his classic Theory of Justice, published in 1971 and further elaborated in subsequent publications, Rawls recognizes that there is no religion or philosophy that can provide a comprehensive view shared by all citizens on how to organize society. He adds that there will possibly never be a single view in any democratic society.

Reasonable people have different beliefs and different views on what is right and what is wrong. Accepting the existence of a "reasonable pluralism," therefore, seems to be a requirement of democratic societies. Furthermore, reasonable people with very different general views can nevertheless identify and expand some common ideas and values—what Rawls calls "an overlapping consensus"—on which to organize societies (Rawls, 2001, p. xvii). Identifying the overlapping consensus for social purposes does not impinge on the liberty of individuals or prevent groups from adhering to and acting within their own comprehensive views of morality. An overlapping consensus, however, allows them to accept that within reasonable limits other persons may act differently, following their own comprehensive views of what is right and wrong.

In order to reach an overlapping consensus, free and equal citizens must agree to engage in a fair system of social cooperation. This requires acceptance that all persons have "the capacity for a sense of justice" and "the capacity to have, to revise, and rationally to pursue a conception of the good" (Rawls 2001, pp 18, 19). In addition, it requires that the social system guarantee the absolute right of each person to an adequate set of basic liberties, such as the freedom to think, to speak, to differ, and to choose individual lifestyles and goals. Of course, there must be some agreed-upon and reasonable limits to freedom and the acceptance of some limited social and economic inequalities, as long as everyone has the right to compete fairly for the social and economic positions within the society.

We quote Rawls not only because we agree with his rejection of present systems—be they capitalist states or social-states—but also because we agree with his assessment that the practical role of political philosophy "is to focus on deeply disputed questions and to see whether, despite appearances, some underlying basis of philosophical and moral agreement can be uncovered. Or, if such a basis of agreement cannot be found, perhaps the divergence of philosophical and moral opinion at the root of divisive political differences can at least be narrowed so that social cooperation on a footing of mutual respect among citizens can still be maintained." To this end, political philosophy must be "realistically utopian," "probing the limits of practicable political possibility" (Rawls, 2001, pp. 2, 4). Utopia is understood as an ideal for which one fights rather than as something that is impossible to achieve.

An important rule for promoting a consensus is to refrain from framing the discussion as a confrontation or as a dilemma. There are occasions when choosing between two options is inevitable, although more frequently other alternative paths exist that may not be readily apparent. Another important rule is to identify the issue, its roots, and its consequences clearly and in all their complexity, based on the best objective evidence available, and to keep up with the latest knowledge and any changes in circumstances (Barzelatto and Dawson, 2003).

Building a consensus is not about denying or ignoring differences or manipulating evidence. It is a process that starts by identifying common views and values and goes on to expand the initial consensus by discussing the roots of the differences. It is a dialogue that requires mutual respect; mere tolerance will not do. Mutual respect means accepting the fact that we may, at least in part, be wrong and that someone else may, at least in part, be right. This attitude requires a strong sense of self-confidence and a solid democratic environment, both of which are indispensable to maintaining the moral integrity of a dialogue that honestly aims to build a sustainable social consensus and not merely at imposing a point of view.

Is an "Overlapping Consensus" on Abortion Possible?

Given the acrimony and the lack of intellectual integrity that characterizes much of the public debate about abortion, reaching an overlapping consensus is at best a very difficult task. Discussing Rawls's notion of overlapping consensus with respect to abortion, two Catholic philosophers, Dombrowski and Deltete, comment that "political liberalism's handling of the abortion debate should result, at the very least, in a modus vivendi but it is also possible that the contending parties might eventually reach an overlapping consensus." (Dombrowski and Deltete, 2000, p. 104) The authors also reveal that one of them is skeptical about the latter possibility, whereas "the other shares Rawls's long-term optimism regarding achieving an overlapping consensus" (Dombrowski and Deltete, 2000, p. 117).

We believe that an overlapping consensus on abortion is possible, having as part of its foundation respect for diversity and the belief that all people are capable of acting as full moral agents. Our optimism is reinforced by the information presented in this book, which we believe incorporates the mainstream of current informed thought and analysis. Particularly inspiring for us—because differences in religious views seem to be the most difficult to overcome—is the consensus reached by prominent theologians at the 1994 interfaith meeting held in Genval and described in Chapter 8. At this meeting, prominent scholars came to agree that given the differences among and within religions and the need to respect religious freedom, no religion could impose its views about abortion on people of other faiths. Furthermore, they condoned decriminalization of abortion as a reasonable move toward decreasing human suffering. As we also saw in Chapter 8, these views on abortion were endorsed in 2004 by an international group of prominent women's rights leaders and distinguished theologians who met in Chiang Mai, Thailand, to discuss women and religion in a globalized world (Center for Health and Social Policy, 2004).

Another inspiring experience came about in response to a tragic event that occurred in Boston on December 30, 1994. A man entered a Planned Parenthood clinic with a rifle, wounded three people, and killed the receptionist. Then he drove two miles to another clinic where legal abortions were performed, shot the receptionist, and wounded another two people. The governor of Massachusetts, William F. Weld, and Boston Cardinal Bernard Law, among others, called for talks among pro-choice and pro-life leaders. Six years later, the *Boston Globe* published an article entitled "Talking with the Enemy," signed by six of the most prominent women in the public debate on abortion in the United States, three of them pro-life and three pro-choice. Their report revealed for the first time that they had been meeting secretly since July 1995 in response to (1) the appeal from the governor and the cardinal and (2) an invitation from Laura Chasin as part of her Public Conversations Project. Attending as individuals rather than as representatives of their organizations, their aim had been not to find common ground or compromise but "to communicate openly"; "to build relationships of mutual respect and understanding; to help deescalate the rhetoric of the abortion controversy; and, of course, to reduce the risk of future shootings" (Fowler et al., 2001, p. F-1). It is fascinating to read how apprehensive, worried, and skeptical these six women and the facilitators were before the first meeting and how difficult the first sessions were. The attendees started by deciding how to refer to each other (the accepted forms for all except one were *pro-life* and *pro-choice*, used in quotation marks) and by identifying hot-button words and phrases that should be avoided (such as *murderers* and *religious fanatics*).

By the first anniversary of the shootings, according to the article signed by the women, "each one of us had come to think differently about those 'on the other side.' . . . As our mutual understanding increased, our respect and affection for one another grew" (Fowler et al., 2001, p. F-1), so much so that two of the pro-lifers attended an anniversary ceremony organized by the pro-choicers. The news media, which had been unaware of the meetings, noted the effect on the way the women spoke in public about the abortion issue.

Although they believed that their differences reflected two irreconcilable world views, the women had met privately for five and a half years (a total of more than 150 hours). During the meetings, they came to see the dignity and goodness in one another, they grew spiritually and intellectually, and they became wiser and more effective leaders. Their purpose in going public was to encourage people to engage in similar dialogues, where "people can disagree frankly and passionately, become clearer in heart and mind about their activism, and at the same time contribute to a more civil and compassionate society" (Fowler et al., 2001, p. F-1).

The Basis for an "Overlapping Consensus" on Abortion

Although people commonly initiate discussions on abortion under the assumption that there are those who are for and those who are against abortion, in truth virtually no one is in favor of abortion per se and virtually no one is against abortion without exception. The public debate has been dominated by two extreme views: one that maintains that women always have the right to decide the fate of the fetus as a part of their bodies and one that maintains that the rights of the fetus, from the time of fertilization, always override the rights of the pregnant woman.

We believe that most people disagree with both of these two extremes and that there is already a narrow but significant overlapping consensus with respect to abortion: (1) Nobody likes the idea of having an abortion or of other people having abortions, but virtually everyone agrees that abortion is morally justified under certain circumstances. (2) There are too many avoidable abortions. (3) Unsafe abortion is a major public health problem. In order to better define and expand this consensus, public debate must focus on how abortions can be prevented and under what circumstances abortion is morally justified.

If we avoid confrontation and unnecessary aggression, it is possible to expand the existing consensus and use it to legislate and regulate abortions while respecting the different value systems of each society. A respectful dialogue would allow (as has been the goal of this book) identification of the depth and extension of the problem, its causes, and its consequences and the interventions that have proven effective in ameliorating the problem.

Taking account of available evidence and the values involved, we propose the following nine points to guide the dialogue that would define a practical consensus and the basic actions that would allow societies to decrease the number of abortions and reduce their negative consequences:

1. There is an unacceptable number of preventable abortions in the world today, and unsafe abortions represent a major public health catastrophe that could be almost completely avoided. Therefore, reducing the number of unwanted pregnancies and abortions and minimizing the human costs of unsafe abortion are desired social goals that will benefit women and society in general. Consequently, societies should promote policies and implement actions that have proven effective in achieving these objectives.

2. *Respect for persons,* including the recognition of and respect for diversity among individuals, is a basic ethical principle and one of the foundations of democracy. It includes freedom of religious belief and respect for diverse faiths as essential components of human social interaction. Consequently, societies that promote a dialogue that seeks to define a practical consensus on abortion should include different value systems, including differing religious perspectives, with the understanding that no religion can impose its values on those who do not profess its faith.

3. Women are human beings with the same rights as men, including the right to make decisions, freely and responsibly, about their sexuality. Nevertheless, societies have traditionally denied equal rights to women and have accepted men's right to impose their sexual decisions on their female partners. This patriarchal culture is a principal cause of unwanted pregnancy, and its passive acceptance is an obstacle to the amelioration of the problem of abortion. Consequently, societies should promote greater gender equity in all spheres of life, including a better balance of power between women and men, which will allow all women the oppor-

tunity to decide when, with whom, and under what circumstances they will pursue their sexual lives. Respecting women's right to true control over their sexual lives is an essential component of these policies and actions.

4. Broad-based, unbiased sexual and reproductive health education, rather than leading to indiscriminate sexual activity, can promote responsible sexual behavior and reduce unwanted pregnancies and induced abortions. Consequently, societies should implement education programs and campaigns based on models that have proven effective in the promotion of responsible sexual behavior and respect between genders.

5. Easy access to effective and safe contraceptive methods through high-quality, user-friendly delivery systems does not promote promiscuity and quite efficiently reduces abortion. Consequently, societies should eliminate all barriers to accessing effective contraceptive methods for all sexually active people.

6. It is not uncommon for women to turn to abortion because they lack family and social support. Consequently, societies should take action to support pregnant women who want to carry a pregnancy to term.

7. Criminalizing abortion and penalizing women who abort does not reduce the number of abortions and—by supporting the market for unsafe, backdoor abortions—greatly increases human suffering and death. Consequently, societies should decriminalize abortion, within socially acceptable limits, and legislate to prevent unwanted pregnancies.

8. When a woman meets the conditions required by the laws of her country to have an abortion, she should have easy access to safe abortion services. Consequently, societies should establish clear guidelines and regulations that will ensure the provision of safe abortion services, free of bureaucratic, economic, or political barriers.

9. Most women have unwanted pregnancies and induced abortions as a result of society's failure to protect their rights. Abortion is typically a decision made as a last resort. Moreover, health facilities have the ethical obligation to treat, without discrimination, all persons who request their services. Consequently, societies must ensure that women who

suffer complications from legal or illegal abortions are treated with full respect and receive health care of the same quality as that provided to any other person who seeks medical help.

Although these views may not, at present, be shared by all groups and, indeed, those holding very extreme views may never agree to all of them, we believe they may come to be acceptable to a vast majority of the world's people. It is not the purpose of this proposal to impose the values of a majority on the views of a minority. It is our goal to find a practical agreement through which societies will be able to address all aspects of abortion and, within reasonable limits, allow women as individuals to follow their conscience in their personal decisions regarding sexuality, reproduction, and abortion.

Some Reflections on the Process for Achieving Consensus

Although we believe that there already exists a general global consensus that too many abortions occur and that unsafe abortion should be eliminated, the same consensus does not exist with respect to which measures should be taken to solve the problem. A major reason for this is that the scientific evidence that demonstrates the effectiveness of specific actions in reducing abortion and its consequences is not readily available to the general public.

The political will to implement the nine points proposed here requires not only clear knowledge of the scientific evidence that supports each point but also broader dissemination of accurate information on the positions of different religious and cultural value systems with respect to abortion—a necessary first step in the process of achieving an overlapping consensus. This information will reveal that the various positions are more tolerant than absolute, thus facilitating a constructive dialogue and expanding the consensus, for example, on which contraceptive methods should be made widely available, who should have access to them, and what information should be included in sex education programs.

We recognize that the process of achieving gender equity may be more difficult and more prolonged because it requires profound cultural change. Nevertheless, improving the balance of power between genders is a clear global trend that, particularly in the more developed parts of the world, has already seen considerable progress. The idea of shared responsibilities between men and women in the pursuit of their sexual and reproductive lives has become increasingly accepted. Thus, it seems logical to incorporate this concept into the growing overlapping consensus.

Virtually no one would argue against support for women who want to carry pregnancy to term. This idea, which is nevertheless rarely included in abortion-related agendas, should therefore be incorporated into the overlapping consensus in order to use public dialogue to ensure that the cultural and legal environment will facilitate the support that women need to carry pregnancies to term and raise their children.

Although the participation of religious groups in building the overlapping consensus may be a challenge, we believe we have shown that the common ground can prevail. The Genval report and the Chiang Mai declaration described in Chapter 8, are convincing examples of agreement among religious leaders on fundamental principles.

The most controversial point in our proposal—the decriminalization of abortion—is one on which there is more agreement than is readily apparent. Reasonable people disagree only with respect to the circumstances under which abortion is morally permissible, but almost everyone agrees that abortion should be legally allowed under certain circumstances. The current controversy concerns conflicting moral value systems, whereas the consensus that we seek involves a practical political approach for addressing the problem of abortion while respecting diverse moral values. Although it implies some cultural change to achieve greater respect for diversity, its concrete focus is a change in legislation, a goal that requires a respectful public dialogue that identifies reasonable restrictions. Solid leadership, to ensure the safety and accessibility of legal abortions for women who meet the legal requirements, is also required. The process of implementing the proposed actions is facilitated by public dialogue that includes collaboration among the medical establishment, women's rights advocacy groups, and the political leadership.

All cultures, including religious and moral systems, are in a constant process of change with respect to the way they apply their fundamental principles under new circumstances. Usually, it is a constructive dialogue that arises from new realities that promotes change in the application of moral values. A resistance to change caused by the uncertainties of the consequences of change is not uncommon. Unfortunately, the natural tendency to interfere with the evolution of constructive dialogue can halt progress. At its worst, this resistance, not infrequently of religious origin, may give rise to extreme responses that have tragic consequences.

The main obstacle to identifying and achieving an overlapping consensus is the existence of extremist positions that oppose change. Extremist views that are not open to respectful discussion cannot be part of the quest to identify an overlapping consensus on which to base a peaceful and just democratic society. Fortunately, extremist positions are in the minority. It is to the great majority that we address this book in the hope that it may contribute toward reducing the human drama of abortion that affects most of us, directly or indirectly, at least once in our lives. The process of seeking and expanding a consensus is a long and hence an urgent one that involves governments, religions, and society at large.

Bibliography

AbouZhar C, Wardlaw T. 2003. Maternal Mortality in 2000: Estimates developed by WHO, UNICEF and UNFPA. Geneva: Department of Reproductive Health and Research (HRP), World Health Organization.

AbouZhar C, Ahman E. 1998. Unsafe abortion and ectopic pregnancy. In: Murray CJL, Lopez AD.(eds.) Health dimensions of sex and reproduction: the global burden of sexually transmitted diseases, HIV, maternal conditions, perinatal disorders, and congenital anomalies. Cambridge, MA, Harvard University. pages 266-296

Adewole IF. 1992. Trends in postabortal mortality and morbidity in Ibadan, Nigeria. Int J Gynaecol Obstet. 38:115–118.

Adler N. 1989. Statement on Behalf of the American Psychological Association before the Human Resources Intergovernmental Relations Subcommittee of the Committee on Governmental Operations, U.S. House of Representatives, March, 16:130–140.

Adler NE, David HP, Major BN, Roth SH, Russo NF, Wyatt GE. 1990. Psychological responses after abortion. Science. 248(4951):41–44.

Ahman E, Shah I. 2002. Unsafe abortion: Worldwide estimates for 2000. Reprod Health Matters. 10(19):13–17.

Alan Guttmacher Institute. 1999. Induced abortion worldwide. Facts in Brief. New York: Alan Guttmacher Institute. Available at: www.guttmacher. org/pubs/fb_0599.pdf.

Albrecht GH. 2003. Contraception and abortion within Protestant Christianity. In: Maguire DC, ed. Sacred Rights: The Case for Contraception and Abortion in World Religions. New York: Oxford University Press, pp 79–103.

Allende S. 1971. Primer Mensaje del Presidente de Chile al país en la inauguración del período ordinario de Sesiones del Congreso Nacional. Santiago: Gobierno de Chile.

Alvarez F, Brache V, Fernandez E, Guerrero B, Guiloff E, Hess R, Salvatierra

AM, Zacharias S. 1988. New insights on the mode of action of intrauterine contraceptive devices in women. Fertil Steril. 49(5):768–773.

Alvarez L. 1992. La regulación de la fecundidad en Cuba. Veracruz: Ministerio de Salud Pública de Cuba.

Alvarez L, Garcia CT, Catasus S, Benitez ME, Martinez MT. 1999. Abortion practice in a municipality of Havana, Cuba. In: Mundigo AI, Indriso C, eds. Abortion in the Developing World. New Delhi: World Health Organization, Vistaar Publications, pp 117–130.

Amaral LH. 2002. Sexo virou bagunça. Revista Veja. 1.741(March 6). Available at: www2.uol.com.br/veja/060302/entrevista.html.

American College of Obstetricians and Gynecologists (ACOG). 2000. ACOG committee opinion: Induction of labor with misoprostol. Int J Gynaecol Obstet. 69(288):77–78.

Araya R, Gómez-Mora H, Vera R, Bastidas JM. 2003. Human spermatozoa motility analysis in a Ringer's solution containing cupric ions. Contraception. 67:161–163.

Atrash HK, MacKay HT, Binkin NJ, CJR Hogue. 1987. Legal abortion in the United States: 1972–1982. Am J Obstet Gynecol. 156:605–612.

Bailey PE, Bruno ZV, Bezerra MF, Queiroz I, Oliveira CM, Chen-Mok M. 2001. Adolescent pregnancy 1 year later: The effects of abortion vs. motherhood in Northeast Brazil. J Adolesc Health. 29:223–232.

Bajos N, Marquet J. 2000. Research on HIV sexual risk: Social relations–based approach in a cross-cultural perspective. Soc Sci Med. 50:1533–1546.

Balaiah D, Naik DD, Parida RC, Ghule M, Hazari KT, Juneja HS. 1999. Contraceptive knowledge, attitude and practices of men in rural Maharashtra. Adv Contracept. 15(3):217–234.

Banerjee N, Sinha A, Kriplani A, Roy KK, Takkar D. 2001. Factors determining the occurrence of unwanted pregnancies. Natl Med J India. 14(4):211–214.

Barker G, Lowenstein I. 1997. Where the boys are: Attitudes related to masculinity, fatherhood, and violence toward women among low-income adolescent and young adult males in Rio de Janeiro, Brazil. Youth and Society. 29(2):166–196.

Barnett W, Freudenberg N, Wille R. 1992. Partnership after induced abortion: A prospective controlled study. Arch Sex Behav. 21(5):443–455.

Barreto T, Campbell OMR, Davies JL, Fauveau V, Filippi VGA, Graham WJ, Mamdani M, Rooney CI, Toubia NF. 1992. Investigating induced abortion in developing countries: Methods and problems. Stud Fam Plann. 23(3):159–170.

Barros A, Santa Cruz A, Sanches N. 1997. Nós fizemos aborto. Revista Veja. 30(37):26–33.

Barzelatto J. 1986. Abortion and its related problems. In: Ratnam SS, Teoh ES, Anandakumar C, eds. Infertility, Male and Female: The Proceedings of the

Twelfth World Congress on Fertility and Sterility, Singapore. Park Ridge, NJ: Parthenon Publishing Group, pp 1–6.

Barzelatto J, Dawson E. 2003. Reproduction and sexuality in a changing world: Reaching consensus. In: Maguire DC, ed. Sacred Rights: The Case for Contraception and Abortion in World Religions. New York: Oxford University Press, pp 255–271.

Battersby S, Chandler JA, Morton MS. 1982. Toxicity and uptake of heavy metals by human spermatozoa. Fertil Steril. 37:230–235.

Baulieu EE. 1985. Contragestion by antiprogestin: A new approach to human fertility control. In: Ciba Foundation, ed. Ciba Foundation Symposium 115. Abortion: Medical Progress and Social Implications. London: Pitman, pp 192–210.

Baulieu EE, Rosenblum M. 1990. The Abortion Pill. New York: Simon and Schuster.

Beauchamp TL, Childress JF. 1994. Principles of Biomedical Ethics, 4th ed. New York: Oxford University Press.

Begum SF. 1993. Saving lives with menstrual regulation. Planned Parenthood Challenges. 1:30–31.

Bengtsson AM, Wahlberg V. 1991. Interruption of pregnancy: Motives, attitudes and contraceptive use. Interviews before abortion, at a family planning clinic, Rome. Gynecol Obstet Invest. 32:139–143.

Bhuiya A, Aziz A, Chowdhury M. 2001. Ordeal of women for induced abortion in a rural area of Bangladesh. J Health Popul Nutr. 19(4): 281–290.

Billings D, Carney XC, Guerreri XR, Muñoz JB, Rivera AS, Chambers V, Voorduim P. 1999. Traditional midwives and postabortion care services in Morelos, Mexico. In: Huntington D, Piet-Pelon NJ, eds. Postabortion Care: Lessons from Operations Research. New York: Population Council, 159–177.

Billy JO, Landale NS, McLaughlin SD. 1986. The effect of marital status at first birth on marital dissolution among adolescent mothers. Demography. 23(3):329–349.

Boonstra H. 2002a. Teen pregnancy: Trends and lessons learned. Issues in Brief. New York: Alan Guttmacher Institute, (1):1–4. Available at: www.guttmacher.org/pubs/ib_1-02.pdf

———— 2002b. Legislators craft alternative vision of sex education to counter abstinence-only drive. Alan Guttmacher Report on Public Policy. 5(2):1–3.

Brazelton TB, Cramer BG. 1990. The earliest relationship: Parents, infants and the drama of early attachment. Readings, Mass: Addison-Wesley Publishing.

Brewer C. 1977. Incidence of post-abortion psychosis: A prospective study. Br Med J. 1(6059):476–477.

Broder DS. 2002. Bush administration's compromise will cost lives. St. Petersburg Times. July 28, p. D-3.

Bromham DR, Oloto EJ. 1997. Tryng to prevent abortion. Eur J Contracept Reprod Health Care. 2(2):81–87.

Buckshee K. 1997. Impact of roles of women on health in India. Int J Gynaecol Obstet. 58:35–42.

Bugalho A, Mocumbi S, Faúndes A, David E. 2000. Termination of pregnancies of less than 6 weeks' gestation with a single dose of 800 µg of vaginal misoprostol. Contraception. 61:47–50.

Bugalho A. 1995. Perfil epidemiológico, complicações e custo do aborto clandestino comparação com aborto hospitalar e parto, em Maputo, Moçambique. PhD diss, Faculty of Medical Sciences, Universidade Estadual de Campinas, Campinas, Brazil.

Butler C. 1996. Late psychological sequelae of abortion: Questions from a primary care perspective. J Fam Pract. 43(4):396–401.

Callahan D. 1970. Abortion: Law, Choice and Morality. New York: Macmillan Publishing, pp. 422–426.

Camacho VH, Murillo AG, Paz M, André R, Simmons R, Young AM, Machicao X, Bahamondes L, Makuch MY, Castro MD, Díaz J, Skibiak J. 1996. Expandiendo opciones de planificación familiar: Diagnóstico cualitativo de la atención en salud reproductiva en Bolivia. Secretaría Nacional de Salud. Ministerio de Desarrollo Humano de Bolívia. Geneva: World Health Organization.

Carbonell Esteve JLL, Varela L, Velazco A, Tanda R, Cabezas E, Sánchez C. 1999. Early abortion with 800 µg of misoprostol by the vaginal route. Contraception. 59:219–225.

Casas L. 1996. Mujeres procesadas por aborto. Santiago, Chile: Foro Abierto de Salud y Derechos Reproductivos.

Castaneda X, Garcia C, Langer A. 1996. Ethnography of fertility and menstruation in rural Mexico. Soc Sci Med. 42(1):133–140.

Cates W, Grimes DA, Schulz KF. 2003. The public health impact of legal abortion: Thirty years later. Perspect Sex Reprod Health. 35:25–28.

Cates W, Grimes DA, Smith JC, Tyler CW. 1977. Legal abortion mortality in the United States: Epidemiologic surveillance, 1972–1974. JAMA. 237:452–455.

Catholics for a Free Choice. 2002. The facts about Catholic health care. Catholic Health Care Update. July:1–3. Available at: www.catholicsforchoice.org/onlinepubs/healthcare/healthcareupdate2002.pdf.

Center for Health and Social Policy. 2004. Women and Religion in a Globalized World: A Conversation of Women's and Religious Leaders. San Francisco. Available at: www.chsp.org/Women_and_Religion_in_a_Globalized_World.pdf.

Center for Reproductive Rights. 2003. The World's Abortion Laws, 2003. New York: Wall Chart.

Chang MC. 1984. The meaning of sperm capacitation: A historical perspective. J Androl. 5:45–50.

Chhabra R. 1996. Abortion in India: An overview. Demography India. 25(1):83–92.

Chi IC. 1991. An evaluation of the Levonorgestrel-releasing IUD: Its advantages and disadvantages when compared to the copper-releasing IUDs. Contraception. 44:573–588.

Chiarotti S, Jurado MG, Aucía A, Arminchiardi S. 2003. Con todo el aire. Report on human rights concerning reproductive health care in public hospitals. Instituto de Genero, Derecho y Desarrollo (INGESNAR), November, Buenos Aires.

Cohen SA. 2002. Elections make drive for reproductive health and rights an even steeper uphill battle. Alan Guttmacher Report on Public Policy. 5(5):1–2, 14.

Colás OR, Andalaft Neto, J, Rosas CF, Kater JR, Pereira IG. 1994. Aborto legal por estupro: Primeiro programa público do país. Bioética. 2:81–85.

Cook RJ. 2000. Developments in Abortion Laws: Comparative and International Perspectives. Ann NY Acad Sci. 913:74–87.

Cook RJ, Dickens BM. 1999. Human rights and abortion laws. Int J Gynaecol Obstet. 65:81–87.

Cook RJ, Maine D. 1987. Spousal veto over family planning services. Am J Public Health. 77(3):339–344.

Costa RG, Hardy E, Osis MJD, Faúndes A. 1995. A decisão de abortar: Processo e sentimentos envolvidos. Cad Saúde Públ (Rio de Janeiro). 11(1):97–105.

Costa SH, Martin IR, Freitas SRS, Pinto CS. 1990. Family planning among low-income women in Rio de Janeiro: 1984–1985. Int Fam Plann Perspect. 16(1):16–22, 28.

Crosby RA, Yarber WL. 2001. Perceived versus actual knowledge about correct condom use among U.S. adolescents: Results from a national study. J Adolesc Health. 28(5):415–420.

Croxatto HB. 2002a. Physiology of gamete and embryo transport through the fallopian tube. Reprod Biomed Online. 4(2):160–169.

————. 2002b. Emergency contraceptive pills: How do they work? IPPF Med Bull. 36(6):1–2.

Croxatto HB, Brache V, Pavez M, Cochon L, Forcelledo ML, Alvarez F, Massai R, Faúndes A, Salvatierra AM. Pituitary-ovarian function following the standard levonorgestrel emergency contraceptive dose or a single 0.75-mg dose given on the days preceding ovulation. 2004. Contraception. 70:442–450.

Croxatto HB, Devoto L, Durand M, Ezcurra E, Larrea F, Nagle C, Ortiz ME,

Vantman D, Vega M, Von Hertzen H. 2001. Mechanism of action of hormonal preparations used for emergency contraception: A review of the literature. Contraception. 63:111–121.

Croxatto HB, Makarainen L. 1998. The pharmakodynamics and efficacy of implanon: An overview of the data. Contraception. 58:91S–97S.

Cumming DC, Cumming CE, Kieren DK. 1991. Menstrual mythology and sources of information about menstruation. Am J Obstet Gynecol. 164(2):472–476.

Dagg PK. 1991. The psychological sequelae of therapeutic abortion—denied and completed. Am J Psychiatry. 148(5):578–585.

Daily Record Debate. 2002. Should DIY abortion pill be allowed? Accessed July 9. Available at: www.dailyrecord.co.uk/printable_version. cfm?objectid= 12017754&siteid=89488.

David HP. 1982. Eastern Europe: Pronatalist policies and private behavior. Popul Bull. 36(6):3-47.

David HP, Dytrych Z, Matejcek Z, Schüller V. 1988. Born Unwanted: Developmental Effects of Denied Abortion. Prague: Avicenum, Czechoslovak Medical Press.

David HP, Friedman HL, van der Tak J, Sevilla MJ. 1978. Transnational trends: An overview. In: Davis HP, Friedman HL, van der Tak J, Sevilla MJ, eds. Abortion in Psychosocial Perspective. New York: Springer Publishing. 3-10.

Dawson DA. 1986. The effects of sex education on adolescent behavior. Fam Plann Perspect. 18(4):162–170.

Demographic and Health Surveys. 2002. Obtaining Data: Survey Indicators STAT compiler. Available at: www.measuredhs.com/data/indicators.

Diallo FS, Traore M, Diakite S, Perrotin F, Dembele F, Diarra I, Dolo A. 2000. Complications of illegal induced abortions at Bamako (Mali) between December 1997 and November 1998. Sante. 10(4):243–247.

Díaz S, Croxatto HB. 2003. Anticoncepción de emergencia. In: Alfredo Pérez-Sánchez, ed. Ginecología, 3rd ed. Santiago, Chile: Publicaciones Técnicas Mediterráneo. 1067–1073.

Dombrowski DA, Deltete R. 2000. A Brief, liberal, Catholic defense of abortion. Chicago: University of Illinois Press, 158p.

Doran DA. 2002. Stoning sentences in Nigeria. Boston Sunday Globe. September 15:A9.

Dougherty J. 2001. Fighting abortion attitudes in Russia. Moscow: CNN, January 21. Available at: www.cdi.org/russia/johnson/5041.html#5.

Duggan P. 2002. A question of choice. Washington Post. April 21 (Part F):1, 3.

Durand M, Cravioto MC, Raymond EG, Durán-Sánchez O, Cruz-Hinojosa ML, Castell-Rodríguez A, Schiavon R, Larrea F. 2001. On the mechanisms of action of short-term levonorgestrel administration in emergency contraception. Contraception. 64:227–234.

Edelman DA, Brenner WE, Berger GS. 1974. The effectiveness and complications of abortion by dilatation and vacuum aspiration versus dilatation and rigid metal curettage. Am J Obstet Gynecol. 119(4):473–480.

Editorial. 2003. The war against women. New York Times. January 12.

Eggleston E, Jackson J, Rountree W, Pan Z. 2000. Evaluation of a sexuality education program for young adolescents in Jamaica. Rev Panam Salud Pública. 7(2):102–112.

Ehrenfeld N. 1999. Female adolescents at the crossroads: Sexuality, contraception and abortion in Mexico. In: Mundigo AI, Indriso C, eds. Abortion in the Developing World. New Delhi, India: World Health Organization, Vistaar Publications, pp 368–386.

Elu MC. 1999. Between political debate and women's suffering: Abortion in Mexico. In: Mundigo AI, Indriso C, eds. Abortion in the Developing World. New Delhi, World Health Organization, Vistaar Publications, pp 245–258.

Ethiopian Society of Obstetrics and Gynecology. 2000. A data base on abortion: Literature review. Addis Ababa, Ethiopia, October.

Ezeh AC. 1993. The influence of spouses over each other's contraceptive attitudes in Ghana. Stud Fam Plann. 24(3):163–174.

Faria VE, Potter JE. 1999. Television, telenovelas, and fertility change in North-East Brazil. In: Leete R. Dynamic of Values in Fertility Change. New York: Oxford University Press, pp 252–272.

Faúndes A, Duarte GA, Andalaft-Neto J, Sousa MH 2004. The closer you are, the better you understand: The reaction of Brazilian Obstetrician-Gynaecologists to unwanted pregnancy. Reproductive Health Matters, 12(24 Supplement): 47–56.

Faúndes A, Hardy E. 1978. Contraception and abortion services at Barros-Luco Hospital: Santiago, Chile. In: David HP, Van de Tak J, Sevilla MJ, eds. Abortion in Psychological Perspective. New York: Springer Publishing, pp 284–297.

Faúndes A, Hardy E, Osis MJ, Duarte G. 2000. O risco para queixas ginecológicas e disfunções sexuais segundo história de violência sexual. Revista Brasileira de Ginecologia e Obstetrícia (RBGO). 22(3):153–157.

Faúndes A, Leocádio E, Andalaft-Neto J. 2002. Making legal abortion accessible in Brazil. Reprod Health Matters. 10(19):120–127.

Faúndes A, Rodrigues G, Hardy E, Mozo RA. 1971. Evaluación de los efectos de un programa de planificación familiar sobre la fecundidad, en una población marginal de Santiago, Chile. Cuadernos Médicos-Sociales. 1:5–16.

Faúndes A, Rodrigues-Galant G, Avendaño O. 1968. The San Gregorio experimental family planning program: Changes observed in fertility and abortion rates. Demography. 5(2):836–845.

Faúndes A, Torres JHR. 2002. O abortamento por risco de vida da mãe. In: Aborto legal: Implicações éticas e religiosas. Seminário Nacional de Intercâmbio e Formação sobre Questões Ético-Religiosas para Técnicos/as dos Programas de Aborto Legal. São Paulo, Brazil: Cadernos Católicas pelo Direito de Decidir, pp 147–158.

Ford NM. 1988. When Did I Begin? Conception of the Human Individual in History, Philosophy and Science. Cambridge, England: Cambridge University Press.

Fortney JA. 1981. The use of hospital resources to treat incomplete abortions: Examples from Latin America. Public Health Rep. 96(6):574–579.

Fowler A, Gamble NN, Hogan FX, Kogut M, McComish M, Thorp B. 2001. Talking with the enemy. Boston Globe, January 28. Available at: http://pubpages.unh.edu/~jds/BostonGlobe.htm

Furstenberg FF Jr, Brooks-Gunn J, Chase-Lansdale L. 1989. Teenaged pregnancy and childbearing. Am Psychol. 44(2):313–320.

Gibbs N. 1991. Teens: The rising risk of AIDS. Time. September 2:56–58.

Gleick E, County B. 1996. No way out. Time. December 23, 148(28):12–15.

Gold RB. 2002. Hierarchy crackdown clouds future of sterilization, EC provision at Catholic Hospitals. Alan Guttmacher Report on Public Policy. 5(2):11,12, 14.

Golding JM, Wilsnack SC, Learman LE. 1998. Prevalence of sexual assault history among women with common gynecologic symptoms. Am J Obstet Gynecol. 179(4):1013–1019.

González DLA, Salinas AAU. 2000. Resultados de una encuesta sobre aborto aplicada a residentes de la especialidad en ginecología y obstetricia en hospitales públicos de la Ciudad de México. Reporte de Investigación del Proyecto "Atención del Aborto en México: Una aproximación a las actitudes de los Médicos." Universidad Autónoma Metropolitana Xochimilco, Xochimilco, Mexico, October.

Goodkind D. 1994. Abortion in Vietnam: Measurements, puzzles and concerns. Stud Fam Plann. 25(6):342–352.

Greene, MF, Ecker, JL. 2004. Abortion, health, and the law. N Engl J Med. 350(2):184–186.

Greenslade FC, Benson J, Winkler J, Henderson V, Wolf M, Leonard A. 1993. Summary of clinical and programmatic experience with manual vacuum aspiration. IPAS (Carrboro, NC). 3(2):1–4.

Grunseit A. 1997. Impacto de la educación en materia de salud sexual y VIH sobre el comportamiento sexual de los jóvenes: Actualización de un análisis. Geneva: Programa Conjunto de las Naciones Unidas sobre VIH/SIDA (ONUSIDA).

Grunseit A, Kippax S, Aggleton P, Baldo M, Slutkin G. 1997. Sexuality education and young people's sexual behavior: A review of studies. J Adolesc Res. 12(4):421–453.

Gudorf CE. 1998. Historical, theological and modern influences on religious treatments of abortion. Presentation at the Advanced Leadership Program for High Officials of the State Family Planning Commission of China. Sponsored by the Center for Health and Social Policy and the Public Media Center, Princeton University, Princeton, NJ, USA, November 1-7.

————. 2003. Contraception and abortion in Roman Catholicism. In: Maguire DC, ed. Sacred Rights: The Case for Contraception and Abortion in World Religions. New York: Oxford University Press, pp 55–78.

Gupte M, Bandewar S, Pisal H. 1997. Abortion needs of women in India: A case study of rural Maharashtra. Reprod Health Matters. 9:77–86.

Handy JA. 1982. Psychological and social aspects of induced abortion. Br J Clin Psychol. 21(1):29–41.

Hardy E, Herud K. 1975. Effectiveness of a contraceptive education program for postabortion patients in Chile. Stud Fam Plann. 6(7):188–191.

Hardy E, Rebello I, Faúndes A. 1993. Aborto entre alunas e funcionárias de uma universidade brasileira. Rev Saúde Pública. 27(2):113–116.

Hardy E, Soza M, Cabezas E, Faúndes A. 1990. Abortion in Cuba, 1989. Annual Meeting of the Population Association of America, Toronto, May 3–5.

Harris G. 2004. Morning-after-pill ruling defies norm. The New York Times, May 8.

Hart G, Macharper T. 1986. Clinical aspects of induced abortion in South Australia from 1970 to 1984. Aust NZ J Obstet Gynaecol. 26(3):219–224.

Heise LL, Pitanguy J, Germain A. 1994. Violence against women: The hidden health burden. World Bank Discussion Papers, Washington, DC, July, 1994 p. 72.

Henshaw SK. 1998. Abortion incidence and services in the United States, 1995–1996. Int Fam Plann Perspect. 30(6):263–270, 287.

Henshaw SK, Finer LB. 2003. The accessibility of abortion services in the United States, 2001. Perspect Sex Reprod Health. 35:16–24.

Henshaw SK, Singh S, Haas T. 1999. The incidence of abortion worldwide. Int Fam Plann Perspect. 25(Suppl):30–38.

Henshaw SK, Singh S, Oye-Adeniran BA, Adewole IF, Iwere N, Cuca YP. 1998. The incidence of induced abortion in Nigeria. Int Fam Plann Perspect. 24(4):156–164.

Henshaw SK, Wallisch LS. 1984. The Medicaid cutoff and abortion services for the poor. Int Fam Plann Perspect. 16(4):171–172, 177–180.

His Holiness the XIV Dalai Lama. 2001. The Art of Living. Hong Kong: Thorsons Printing Press. 176p.

Hollander D. 1995. Mifepristone and vaginal misoprostol are effective, acceptable and inexpensive medical abortion regime. Fam Plann Perspect. 27(5):223–224.

Holmes KK, Levine R, Weaver M. Effectiveness of condoms in preventing sexually transmitted infections. Bull World Health Organ. 2004 Jun;82(6):454-61.

Huntington D, Nawar L, Abdel-Hady D. 1997. Women's perceptions of abortion in Egypt. Reprod Health Matters. 9:101–107.

Huntington D, Nawar L, Hassan EO, Youssef H, Abdel-Tawab N. 1998. The postabortion caseload in Egyptian hospitals: A descriptive study. Int Fam Plann Perspect. 24(1):25–31.

Ignatieff M. 2001. The attack on human rights. Foreign Affairs. 80:102–116. Available at: www.foreignaffairs.org/20011101faessay5777/michael-ignatieff/the-attack-on-human-rights.html

Indian Council of Medical Research, Task Force on Natural Family Planning. 1996. Field trial of Billings ovulation method of natural family planning. Contraception. 53:69–74.

Irwin CE. 2004. Adolescent sexuality and reproductive health: Where are we in 2004? J Adolesc Health. 34:353–355.

Isaacs SL, Sanhueza H. 1975. Induced abortion in Latin America: The legal perspective. In: Pan American Health Organization, ed. Epidemiology of abortion and practices of fertility regulation in Latin America: Selected reports. Washington, DC: Pan American Health Organization, (Scientific Publication 36) p.39-49.

Jagannathan R. 2001. Relying on surveys to understand abortion behavior: Some cautionary evidence. Am J Public Health. 91(11):1825–1831.

Jain JK, Meckstroth KR, Mishell DR Jr. 1999. Early pregnancy termination with intravaginally administered sodium chloride solution-moistened misoprostol tablets: Historical comparison with mifepristone and oral misoprostol. Am J Obstet Gynecol. 181:1386–1391.

Jain JK, Dutton C, Harwood B, Meckstroth K, Mishell DR Jr. 2002. A prospective randomized, double-blinded, placebo-controlled trial comparing mifepristone and vaginal misoprostol to vaginal misoprostol alone for elective termination of early pregnancy. Hum Reprod. 17:1477–1482.

Jain S. 2003. The right to family planning, contraception and abortion: The Hindu view. In: Maguire DC, ed. Sacred Rights: The Case for Contraception and Abortion in World Religions. New York: Oxford University Press, pp 129–143.

JAMA. 1992. The myth of the abortion trauma syndrome [commentary]. JAMA. 268(15):2078–2079.

Jecht EW, Bernstein GS. 1973. The influence of copper on the motility of human spermatozoa. Contraception. 7(5):381–401.

Jewkes R, Vundule C, Maforah F, Jordaan E. 2001. Relationship dynamics and teenage pregnancy in South Africa. Soc Sci Med. 52:733–744.

Johansson E, Brache V, Alvarez F, Faúndes A, Cochon L, Ranta S, Lovern M, Kumar N. 2002. Pharmacokinetic study of different dosing regimens of levonorgestrel for emergency contraception in healthy women. Hum Reprod. 17(6):1472–1476.

Johns Hopkins Center for Communication Programs. 2001. Nicaraguan youth begin to play it safe Communication Impact: November, 12:1-2

Jones RK, Darroch JE, Henshaw SK. 2002. Patterns in the socioeconomic characteristics of women obtaining abortion in 2000 to 2001. Perspect Sex Reprod Health. 34(5):226–235.

Justesen A, Kapiga SH, van Asten HAGA. 1992. Abortions in a hospital setting: Hidden realities in Dar es Salaam, Tanzania. Stud Fam Plann. 23(5):325–329.

Kabir SM. 1989. Causes and consequences of unwanted pregnancy from Asian women's perspectives. Int J Gynaecol Obstet. Suppl. 3:9-14.

Karim SMM. 1971. Once-a-month vaginal administration of prostaglandins E2 and F2alfa for fertility control. Contraception. 3(3):173–183.

Karim SMM, Filshie GM. 1970a. Therapeutic abortion using prostaglandin F2alfa. Lancet. 1:157–159.

————. 1970b. Use of prostaglandin E2 for therapeutic abortion. Br Med J. 3:198–200.

Kaufman J. 1993. The cost of IUD failure in China. Stud Fam Plann. 24(3):194–196.

Kennedy KI, Visness CM. 1992. Contraceptive efficacy of lactational amenorrhoea. Lancet. 339:227–230.

Kero A, Lalos A. 2000. Ambivalence—a logical response to legal abortion: A prospective study among women and men. J Psychosom Obstet Gynaecol. 21(2):81–91.

Kero A, Lalos A, Högberg U, Jacobsson L. 1999. The male partner involved in legal abortion. Hum Reprod. 14(10):2669–2675.

Ketting E, Visser AP. 1994. Contraception in the Netherlands: The low abortion rate explained. Patient Educ Couns. 23(3):161–171.

Khan ME, Barge S, Philip G. 1996. Abortion in India - an overview. Social Change. Sept-Dec, 26(3 & 4): 208-225.

Kirby D. 2001. Emerging Answers: Research Findings on Programs to Reduce Teen Pregnancy. Washington, DC: National Campaign to Prevent Teen Pregnancy.

Kirby D, Resnick MD, Downes B, Kocher T, Gunderson P, Potthoff S, Zelterman D, Blum RW. 1993. The effects of school-based health clinics in St. Paul on school-wide birthrates. Fam Plann Perspect. 25(1):12–16.

Kitchen WH, Rickards AL, Ford GW, Ryan MM, Lissenden JV. 1985. Liveborn infants of 24 to 28 weeks' gestation: Survival and sequelae at two years of age. In: Ciba Foundation Symposium 115. Abortion: Medical Progress and Social Implications. London: Pitman, pp 122–135.

Koch UJ, Vogel M. 1979. Effects of ML Cu250 on endometrium and sperm migration. In: Hafez ESE, Van Os WAA, eds. Medicated IUDs and

Polymeric Delivery Systems: Proceedings of the International Symposium. Amsterdam, Holland, June 27-30. Detroit, Michigan: Hafez and Van Os: pp 21A–B.

Konje JC, Obisesan KA, Ladipo AO. 1992. Health and economic consequences of septic induced abortion. Int J Gynaecol Obstet. 37(3):193–197.

Ladipo OA. 1989. Preventing and managing complications of induced abortion in Third World countries. Int J Gynaecol Obstet. 3(Suppl):21–28.

Lane SD, Jok JM, El-Mouelhy MT. 1998. Buying safety: The economics of reproductive risk and abortion in Egypt. Soc Sci Med. 47(8):1089–1099.

Langer A, Garcia-Barrios C, Heimburger A, Campero L, Stein K, Winikoff B, Barahona V. 1999. Improving postabortion care with limited resources in a public hospital in Oaxaca, Mexico. In: Huntington D, Piet-Pelon NJ, eds. Postabortion Care: Lessons from Operations Research. New York: Population Council, pp 80–101.

Larsson B, Hamberger L. 1977. The concentration of copper in human uterine secretion during four years after insertion of a copper-containing intrauterine device. Fertil Steril. 28(6):624–626.

Lawson HW, Frye A, Atrash HK, Smith JC, Shulman HB, Ramick M. 1994. Abortion mortality, United States, 1972 through 1987. Am J Obstet Gynecol. 171(5):1365–1372.

Lazarus ES. 1997. Politicizing abortion: Personal morality and professional responsibility of residents training in the United States. Soc Sci Med. 44(9):1417–1425.

Lewis PR, Brown JB, Renfree MB, Short RV. 1991. The resumption of ovulation and menstruation in a well-nourished population of women breastfeeding for an extended period of time. Fertil Steril. 55(3):529–536.

Liskin LS. 1992. Maternal morbidity in developing countries: A review and comments. Int J Gynaecol Obstet. 37(2):77–87.

Loy DR. 2002. On the Nonduality of Good and Evil: Buddhist Reflections on the New Holy War. In: Piven JS, Ziolo P, and Lawton HW, eds. Terror and Apocalypse. Psychological Undercurrents of History, volume II, New York: Writer's Showcase, pp. 244-267.

Lumley J. 1980. The image of the fetus in the first trimester. Birth Fam J. 7:5–14.

Machel JZ. 2001. Unsafe sexual behaviour among schoolgirls in Mozambique: A matter of gender and class. Reprod Health Matters. 9(17):82–90.

Macklin R. 1999. Against Relativism: Cultural Diversity and the Search for Ethical Universals in Medicine. New York: Oxford University Press.

Maforah F, Wood K, Jewkes R. 1997. Backstreet abortion: Women's experiences. Curationis. 20(2):79–82.

Maguire DC. 2001. Sacred Choices: The Right to Contraception and Abortion in Ten World Religions. Minneapolis: Fortress Press.

Maguire, DC, ed. 2003. Sacred Rights: The Case for Contraception and Abortion in World Religions. New York: Oxford University Press.

Maine D. 1981. Family Planning: Its Impact on the Health of Women and Children. New York: Columbia University, Center for Population and Family Health.

Major B, Richards C, Cooper ML, Cozzarelli C, Zubek J. 1998. Personal resilience, cognitive appraisals, and coping: An integrative model of adjustment to abortion. J Pers Soc Psychol. 74(3):735–752.

Marions L, Hultenby K, Lindell I, Sun X, Stabi B, Danielsson KG. 2002. Emergency contraception with mifepristone and levonorgestrel: Mechanism of action. Obstet Gynecol. 100(1):65–71.

Marston C, Cleland J. 2003. Relationships between contraception and abortion: A review of the evidence. Int Fam Plann Perspect. 29(1):6–13.

Mashalaba NN. 1989. Commentary on the causes and consequences of unwanted pregnancy from an African perspective. Int J Gynaecol Obstet. Suppl.3:15–19].

Matejcek Z, Dytrych Z, Schüller V. 1985. Follow-up study of children born to women denied abortion. In: Ciba Foundation Symposium 115. Abortion: Medical Progress and Social Implications. London: Pitman, pp 136–149.

Maxwell C, Boyle M. 1995. Risky heterosexual practices amongst women over 30: Gender, power and long term relationships. AIDS Care. 7(3):277–293.

Mbizvo MT, Kasule J, Gupta V, Rusakaniko S, Koniti SN, Mpanju-shumbuschu W, Sebina-zziwa AJ, Mwateba R, Padayachy J. 1997. Effects of a randomized health education intervention on aspects of reproductive health knowledge and reported behaviour among adolescents in Zimbabwe. Soc Sci Med. 44(5):573–577.

McCarthy J, Menken J. 1979. Marriage, remarriage, marital disruption and age at first birth. Fam Plann Perspect. 11(1):21–23, 27–30.

McCauley A, Salter C. 1995. Meeting the needs of young adults. Population Reports, series J, no. 41. Baltimore, Johns Hopkins School of Public Health, Population Information Program, vol. 23(3), October.

McKay HE, Rogo KO, Dixon DB. 2001. FIGO society survey: Acceptance and use of new ethical guidelines regarding induced abortion for non-medical reasons. Int J Gynaecol Obstet. 75:327–336.

Middleman AB. 1999. Review of sexuality education in the United States for health professionals working with adolescents. Curr Opin Pediatr. 11(4):283–286.

Ministerio de Salud Pública de Cuba. 2001. Anuario Estadístico de Salud. Habana, Cuba: Dirección Nacional de Estadística. MINSAP.

Ministério da Saúde do Brasil. 1999. Sistema de Informações Hospitalares do Sistema Único de Saúde. Datasus. Available at: www.datasus.gov.br.

Mishell DR Jr. 1998. Intrauterine devices: Mechanism of action, safety and efficacy. Contraception. 58:45S–53S.

Moore ML. 2000. Adolescent pregnancy rates in three European countries: "Lessons to be learned?" J Obstet Gynecol Neonatal Nurs. 29(4):355–362.

Morowitz HJ, Trefil JS. 1992. The facts of life: Science and the abortion controversy. New York: Oxford University Press.

Munera A. 1994. Problemática religiosa de la mujer que aborta. Report to the Ford Foundation of a presentation to the Encounter of Researchers on Induced Abortions in Latin America and the Caribbean, Universidad Externado de Colombia, Bogotá, 15-18 de Noviembre, 1994.

Nankinga J. 2002. Women activists want legal abortion: New vision, Kampala. Webposted April 25. Available at: http://allafrica.com/stories/printable/200204250278.html.

Nations MK, Misago C, Fonseca W, Correia LL, Campbell OMR. 1997. Women's hidden transcripts about abortion in Brazil. Soc Sci Med. 44(12):1833–1845.

Nikkanen V, Söderstrom KO, Tuusa S, Jaakkola UM. 2000. Effect of local epididymal levonorgestrel on the fertilizing ability of male rat: A model for post-testicular contraception. Contraception. 61:401–406.

Nordic Family Planning Associations (Danish, Icelandic, Finish, Norwegian, Swedish). 1999. The Nordic resolution on adolescent sexual health and rights. Resolution presented at the International Conference on Population and Development (ICPD)+5 Forum, The Hague, February.

Oodit G, Bhowon U. 1999. The use of induced abortion in Mauritius: An alternative to fertility regulation or an emergency procedure? In: Mundigo AI, Indriso C, eds. Abortion in the Developing World. New Delhi, India: World Health Organization, Vistar Publications, pp 151–166.

Ortiz ME, Croxatto HB. 1990. Human eggs in the female genital tract. In: Asch RH, Balmaceda JP, Johnston I, eds. Gamete Physiology: Serono Symposia. Norwell, Mass, pp 173–185.

Ortiz ME, Croxatto HB, Bardin CW. 1996. Mechanisms of action of intrauterine devices. Obstet Gynecol Surv. 51(Suppl [12]):S42–S51.

Ortiz ME, Ortiz RE, Fuentes MA, Parraguez VH, Croxatto HB. 2004. Post-coital administration of levonorgestrel does not interfere with post-fertilization events in the new-world monkey Cebus paella. Hum Reprod. 19(6):1352–1356.

Osis MJD, Duarte GA, Padua KS, Espejo X. 2003. Escolha livre e informada na regulação da fecundidade. Relatório final apresentado à Organização Mundial da Saúde, Cemicamp, Campinas, Brasil, Junho.

Osis MJD, Hardy E, Faúndes A, Alves G, Balarezo G. 1994. Opinião das mulheres sobre as circunstâncias em que os hospitais deveriam fazer abortos. Cad Saúde Publ. 10(3):320–330.

Osis MJD, Hardy E, Faúndes A, Rodrigues T. 1996. Dificuldades para obter informações da população de mulheres sobre aborto ilegal. Rev Saúde Pública. 30(5):444–451.

Overington C. 2002. Bush stalls UN pact on child welfare that "backs abortion." Available at: www.smh.com.au/cgi-bin/common/printArticle. pl?path =/articles/2002.

Oyediran KA, Ishola GP, Adewuyi AA. 2002. Knowledge of possible pregnancy at first coitus: A study of in school adolescents in Ibadan, Nigeria. J Biosoc Sci. 34(2):233–248.

Pachauri S. 2001. Male involvement in reproductive health care. J Indian Med Assoc. 99(3):138–141.

Panos Health and Reproductive Health Reports. 1998. Women's health: Using human rights to gain reproductive rights. Briefing no. 32. December. [London, UK]

Park Ridge Center for the Study of Health, Faith and Ethics. 1994. World religions and the 1994 United Nations Conference on Population and Development: A report on an international and interfaith consultation. Genval, Belgium, and Chicago, Illinois, May 4-7, pp. 1-20.

Payne EC, Kravitz AR, Notman MT, Anderson JV. 1976. Outcome following therapeutic abortion. Arch Gen Psychiatry. 33(6):725–733.

Peltzer K. 2001. Knowledge and practice of condom use among first year students at University of the North, South Africa. Curationis 24(1):53–57.

Peremans L, Hermann I, Avonts D, Van Royen P, Denekens J. 2000. Contraceptive knowledge and expectations by adolescents: An explanation by focus groups. Patient Educ Couns. 40(2):133–141.

Pérez Aguirre LF. 2000. Religious aspects of induced abortions. Paper presented at Meeting of Parliamentarians from Latin America and the Caribbean on Induced Abortion. Santafé de Bogotá: Universidad Externado de Colombia, pp 47–69.

Peyron R, Aubeny E, Targosz V, Silvestre L, Renault M, Elkik F, Leclerc P, Ulmann A, Baulieu EE. 1993. Early termination of pregnancy with mifepristone (RU-486) and the orally active prostaglandin misoprostol. N Engl J Med. 328(21):1509–1513.

Pick de Weiss S, Diaz Loving R, Andrade Palos P, David HP. 1990. Effect of sex education on the sexual and contraceptive practices of female teenagers in Mexico City. J Psychol Hum Sex. 3(2):71–93.

Pitanguy J, Garbayo LS. 1995. Relatório do seminário: A implementação do aborto legal no serviço público de saúde. Rio de Janeiro: Cidadania, Estudo, Pesquisa, Informação e Ação (CEPIA). 96p.

Plaza S, Briones H. 1962. El aborto como problema asistencial. Rev Méd Chil. 91:294–299.

Pope LM, Adler NE, Tschann JM. 2001. Postabortion psychological adjustment: Are minors at increased risk? J Adolesc Health. 29(1):2–11.

Popov AA. 1991. Family planning and induced abortion in the USSR: Basic health and demographic characteristics. Stud Fam Plann. 22(6)368–377.

Population Council. 2001. Reducing HIV infection among youth: What can schools do? Horizons Report, Washington, USA, November.

Potter LS. 1996. How effective are contraceptives? The determination and measurement of pregnancy rates. Obstet Gynecol. 88:13–23.

Ramos S, Gogna M, Petracci M, Romero M, Szulic D. 2001. Los médicos frente a la anticoncepción y el aborto: Una transición ideológica? Buenos Aires, Centro de Estudios de Estado y Sociedad (CEDES).

Rawls J. 2001. Justice as Fairness: A restatement. Kelly E, ed. Cambridge, Mass: Belknap Press of Harvard University, 214p.

Requena M. 1965. Social and economic correlates of induced abortion in Santiago, Chile. Demography. 2:33–49.

———. 1966. Condiciones determinantes del aborto inducido. Rev Méd Chil. 94(11):714–722.

———. 1969. Chilean program of abortion control and fertility planning: Present situation and forecast for the next decade. In: Behrman SJ, Corsa L Jr, Freedman R, eds. Fertility and Family Planning: A World Review. Ann Arbor: University of Michigan Press. 478-489.

Richards A, Lachman E, Pitsoe SB, Moodley J. 1985. The incidence of major abdominal surgery after septic abortion—an indicator of complications due to illegal abortion. S Afr Med J. 68(11):799–800.

Rogers JL, Stoms GB, Phifer JL. 1989. Psychological impact of abortion: Methodological and outcomes summary of empirical research between 1966 and 1988. Health Care Women Int. 10(4):347–376.

Romans-Clarkson SE. 1989. Psychological sequelae of induced abortion. Aust NZ J Psychiatry. 23(4):555–565.

Ros A, Mancaniello L, Amantéa P, Bouche M. 1979. La motilité des spermatozoides dans le mucus cervical chez les porteuses de DIU au cuivre. Contracept Fertil Sex. 7(8):551-556.

Rosselot J, Adriazola G, Avendaño O, Borgoño JM, Faúndes A, Gomez C, Keymer E, Pfau L, Plaza L, Rodriguez F, Ugarte JM. 1966. Informe sobre política del Servicio Nacional de Salud para regular la natalidad en Chile. Rev Méd Chil. 94(11):744–750.

Roth J, Krishnan SP, Bunch E. 2001. Barriers to condom use: Results from a study in Mumbai (Bombay), India. AIDS Educ Prev. 13(1):65–77.

Russo NF, Dabul AJ. 1997. The relationship of abortion to well-being: Do race and religion make a difference? Professional Psychology – Research and Practice. 28(1):23–31.

Sable MR, Libbus MK. 1998. Beliefs concerning contraceptive acquisition and use among low-income women. J Health Care Poor Underserved. 9(3):262–275.

Sachedina Z. 1989. Religion, reproduction and the law: Perspectives from Judaism, Christianity, Islam, Hinduism and Buddhism. Internship Report to the Director of the Special Program of Research, Development and Research Training in Human Reproduction (HRP), World Health Organization, Geneva. March, 1989

Sass HM. 1994. The moral significance of brain-life criteria. In: Beller FK, Weir R, eds. The Beginning of Human Life. Boston: Kluwer Academic Publishers. 57-70.

Sathe AG. 1994. Introduction of sex education in schools: Perceptions of Indian Society. J Fam Welfare. 40(1):30–37.

Schaff EA, Fielding SL, Eisinger SH, Stadalius LS, Fuller L. 2000. Low-dose mifepristone followed by vaginal misoprostol at forty-eight hours for abortion up to sixty-three days. Contraception. 61:41–46.

Schaff EA, Fielding SL, Westhoff C. 2001. Randomized trial of oral versus vaginal misoprostol at one day after mifepristone for early medical abortion. Contraception. 64(2):81–85.

Schenker JG. 1997. Report of the Committee for the Study of Ethical Aspects of Human Reproduction. Ethical aspects in the management of newborn infants at the threshold of viability: Int J Gynaecol Obstet. 59:165–168.

Schenker JG, Cain JM. 1999. International Federation of Gynecology and Obstetrics Committee for the Ethical Aspects of Human Reproduction and Women's Health. Int J Gynaecol Obstet. 64:317–322.

Serour GI. 1994. Islam and the four principles. In: Gillon R, ed. Principles of Health Care Ethics. London: John Wiley and Sons. 75-91.

Shaikh S. 2003. Family planning, contraception and abortion in Islam: Undertaking Khilafah. Moral agency, justice and compassion. In: Maguire DC, ed. Sacred Rights: The Case for Contraception and Abortion in World Religions. New York: Oxford University Press, pp 105–128.

Shang G. 2003. Excess, lack and harmony: Some Confucian and Taoist approaches to family planning and population control. Tradition and the modern challenge. In: Maguire DC, ed. Sacred Rights: The Case for Contraception and Abortion in World Religions. New York: Oxford University Press, pp 217–235.

Silberschmidt M, Rasch V. 2001. Adolescent girls, illegal abortions and "sugar-daddies" in Dar es Salaam: Vulnerable victims and active social agents. Soc Sci Med. 52:1815–1826.

Singh S, Cabigon JV, Hossain A, Kamal H, Perez AE. 1997. Estimating the level of abortion in the Philippines and Bangladesh. Int Fam Plann Perspect. 23:100–107, 144.

Singh S, Darroch JE. 2000. Adolescent pregnancy and childbearing: Levels and trends in developed countries. Fam Plann Perspect. 32(1):14–23.

Singh S, Sedgh G. 1997. Relación del aborto con las tendencias anticonceptivas y de fecundidad en el Brasil, Colombia y México. Perspect Int Plan Fam. Número especial de 1997, págs. 2-13.

Singh S, Wulf D. 1994. Estimated levels of abortion in six Latin American countries. Int Fam Plann Perspect. 20:4–13.

Skjeldestad FE. 1994. When pregnant—why induced abortion? Scand J Soc Med. 22(1):68–73.

————. 1997. Increased number of induced abortions in Norway after media coverage of adverse vascular events from the use of third-generation oral contraceptives. Contraception. 55:11–14.

Sparrow MJ. 1999. Condom failures in women presenting for abortion. NZ Med J. 112(1094):319–321.

Speckhard A, Rue V. 1992. Post-abortion syndrome, a growing health problem. J Soc Issues.. 48(3): 95-119.

Stephen C. 2002. Russians despair as more bodies of newborn babies discovered. Worldbytes News. March 16.

Stephenson P, Wagner M, Badea M, Serbanescu F. 1992. Commentary: The public health consequences of restricted induced abortion. Lessons from Romania. Am J Public Health. 82(10):1328–1331.

Stewart FH, Shields WC, Hwang AC. 2004. Faulty assumptions, harmful consequences: Coming to terms with adolescent sexuality. Contraception. 69:345–346.

Stille A. 2001. New attention for the idea that abortion averts crime. New York Times. April 14.

Sundström K. 1996. Abortion across social and cultural borders. Paper presented at the Seminar on Socio-cultural and Political Aspects of Abortion from an Anthropological Perspective. Trivandrum, India, March 25–28.

Suwanbubba P. 2003. The right to family planning, contraception and abortion in Thai Buddhism. In: Maguire DC, ed. Sacred Rights: The Case for Contraception and Abortion in World Religions. New York: Oxford University Press, pp 145–165.

Tamang AK, Shrestha N, Sharma K. 1999. Determinants of induced abortion and subsequent reproductive behavior among women in three urban districts of Nepal. In: Mundigo AI, Indriso C, eds. Abortion in the Developing World. New Delhi, India: World Health Organization, Vistar Publications, pp 167–190.

Tatum HJ. 1973. Metalic copper as an intrauterine contraceptive agent. Am J Obstet Gynecol. 117(5):602–618.

Tietze C, Lewit S. 1972. Joint Program for the Study of Abortion (JPSA): Early medical complications of legal abortion. Stud Fam Plann. 3(6):97–122.

Tietze C, Pakter J, Berger GS. 1973. Mortality with legal abortion in New York City, 1970–1972. JAMA. 225(5):507–509.

Töpfer-Petersen E, Petrounkina AM, Ekhlasi-Hundrieser M. 2000. Oocyte-sperm interactions. Anim Reprod Sci. 60–61:653–662.

Törnbom M, Ingelhammar E, Lilja H, Möller A, Svanberg B. 1994. Evaluation of stated motives for legal abortion. J Psychosom Obstet Gynaecol. 15(1):27–33.

Törnbom M, Möller A. 1999. Repeat abortion: A qualitative study. J Psychosom Obstet Gynaecol. 20(1):21–30.

Torres A, Forrest JD. 1988. Why do women have abortions? Fam Plann Perspect. 20(4):169–176.

Trussell J. 1998. Contraceptive efficacy. In: Hatcher RA, Trussell J, Stewart F, Cates W Jr, Stewart GK, Guest F, Kowal D, eds. Contraceptive Technology, 17th rev ed. New York: Ardent Media, pp 779–844.

Ulmann A, Silvestre L. 1994. RU486: The French experience. Hum Reprod. 9(Suppl 1):126–130.

Underwood C, Hachonda H, Serlemitsos E, Bharath U. 2001. Impact of the heart campaign. Findings from the Youth Surveys, 1999 and 2000, November. Zambian Integrated Health Program (ZIHP)} Lusaka, Zambia.

United Nations Population Fund UNFPA. 1995. Contraceptive requirements and logistics management needs in Brazil. Technical Report number 21. New York, 1995

United Nations. 1993. Report of the World Conference on Human Rights. Vienna, June 14–25.

————. 1995a. Report of the International Conference on Population and Development. Cairo, September 5–13. New York, March, 100p.

————. 1995b. Report of the Fourth World Conference on Women. Beijing, September 4–15.

————. Population Division. 1999. United Nations, Population Division, wall chart, publication ST/ESA/SER.A/178, New York, also available at www.un.org/esa/population/publications/abt/abtnote.htm

————. 2001a. Abortion policies. A global review. Vol 1. New York.

————. 2001b. Abortion policies. A global review. Vol 2. New York.

————. 2002. Abortion policies. A global review. Vol 3. New York.

Viel B. 1985. Induced abortion in Latin America: Impact on health. Symposium to honor Cristopher Tietze, Berlin, September 21-22.

Vilar D. 2002. Abortion: The Portuguese case. Reprod Health Matters. 10(19):156–161.

von Hertzen H, Piaggio G, Ding J, Chen J, Song S, Bártfai G, Ng E, Gemzell-Danielsson K, Oyunbileg A, Wu S, Cheng W, Lúdicke F, Pretnar-Darovec A, Kirkman R, Mittal S, Khomassuridze A, Apter D, Peregoudov A. 2002. Low dose mifepristone and two regimens of levonorgestrel for emergency contraception: A WHO multicentre randomized trial. Lancet. 360:1803–1810.

Weller S, Davis K. 2002. Condom effectiveness in reducing heterosexual HIV transmission. Cochrane Database Syst Rev. (1):CD003255.

Wilcox AJ, Weinberg CR, Baird DD. 1995. Timing of sexual intercourse in relation to ovulation: Effects on the probability of conception, survival of the pregnancy, and sex of the baby. N Engl J Med. 333(23):1517–1521.

————. 1998. Post-ovulatory aging of the human oocyte and embryo failure. Hum Reprod. 13(2):394–397.

Winkler J, Oliveras E, McIntosh N. 1995. Postabortion care. A reference manual for improving quality of care: Postabortion Care Consortium (AVSC International, Ipas, IPPF, JHU/CCP, JHPIEGO, Pathfinder International), Baltimore.

Wong KS, Ngai CSW, Wong AYK, Tang LCH, Ho PC. 1998. Vaginal misoprostol compared with vaginal gemeprost in termination of second trimester pregnancy. Contraception. 58:207–210.

World Health Organization (WHO). 1977. Recommended definitions, terminology and format for statistical tables related to the perinatal period and use of a new certificate for cause of perinatal deaths: Modifications recommended by FIGO as amended October 14, 1976. Acta Obstet Gynecol Scand. 56(3):247–253.

————. 1981. A prospective multicentre trial of the ovulation method of natural family planning. II: The effectiveness phase. Fertil Steril. 36(5):591–598.

————. 1992. The prevention and management of unsafe abortion. Report of a technical working group, World Health Organization (WHO/MSM/92.5), Geneva. April 12-15.

————. 1993. Abortion: A Tabulation of Available Data on the Frequency and Mortality of Unsafe Abortion, 2nd ed. Geneva: World Health Organization, Division of Family Health.

————. 1995. Complications of Abortion: Technical and Managerial Guidelines for Prevention and Treatment. Geneva: World Health Organization.

————. 1997. Unsafe Abortion: Global and Regional Estimates of Incidence of and Mortality Due to Unsafe Abortion with a Listing of Available Country Data, 3rd ed. Geneva: World Health Organization, Division of Reproductive Health (Technical Support).

————. Task Force on Postovulatory Methods of Fertility Regulation. 1998. Randomised controlled trial of levonorgestrel versus the Yuzpe regimen of combined oral contraceptives for emergency contraception. Lancet. 352:428–433.

————, Task Force on Postovulatory Methods of Fertility Regulation. 2000. Comparison of two doses of mifepristone in combination with misoprostol for early medical termination: A randomized trial. Br J Obstet Gynaecol. 107:524–530.

————. 2004. Unsafe Abortion: Global and Regional Estimates of Incidence of Unsafe Abortion and Associated Mortality in 2000, 4th ed. Geneva: World Health Organization.

Yao M, Tulandi T. 1997. Current status of surgical and nonsurgical management of ectopic pregnancy. Fertil Steril. 67(3):421–433.

Zheng Z, Zhou Y, Zheng L, Yang Y, Zhao D, Lou C, Zhao S. 2001. Sexual behavior and contraceptive use among unmarried, young women migrant workers in five cities in China. Reprod Health Matters. 9(17):118–127.

Zipper J, Delgado R, Guiloff E. 1963. Estudios experimentales del mecanismo de acción de cuerpos intrauterinos. Rev Chil Obstet Ginecol. 28:18–22.

Zipper J, Medel M, Prager R. 1969. Suppression of fertility by intrauterine copper and zinc in rabbits: A new approach to intrauterine contraception. Am J Obstet Gynecol. 105(4):529–534.

Zolese G, Blacker CV. 1992. The psychological complications of therapeutic abortion. Br J Psychiatry. 160:742–749.

Zoloth L. 2003. Each one an entire world: A Jewish perspective in family planning. In: Maguire DC, ed. Sacred Rights: The Case for Contraception and Abortion in World Religions. New York: Oxford University Press, pp.21-53.

Index

About the Authors

Aníbal Faúndes was born in Chile. He graduated from medical school in April 1955 and became a full professor of obstetrics at the Universidad de Chile in 1970. He was coordinator of the Women's Health Program during the first year of President Salvador Allende's government, was forced to leave Chile after Augusto Pinochet's military coup in 1973, and subsequently became an advisor in maternal health and family planning for the government of the Dominican Republic.

In 1976 he took a position as professor of obstetrics at the State University of Campinas, in São Paulo, Brazil. In 1977, along with Professor José A. Pinotti, he created the Center for Research in Maternal and Neonatal Health (Cemicamp)—now known as the Center for Research in Reproductive Health—which he chaired until 2003. Since 1996 he has organized—in collaboration with a number of institutions—the annual Inter-professional Forum on Sexual Violence. He has received international recognition as chair of the Committee on Resources for Research for the World Health Organization's Human Reproduction Program, as vice president of the Board of Directors of the International Women's Health Coalition of New York, as president of the Latin American Association of Investigators in Human Reproduction (ALIRH), and as president of the International Association for Maternal and Neonatal Health (IAMANEH). Currently, he chairs the Committee on Sexual and Reproductive Rights of the International Federation of Gynecology and Obstetrics (FIGO).

Aníbal Faúndes has authored more than 370 articles published in scientific journals; edited several books; and, most recently, translated into English—with José Barzelatto—this edition of *The Human Drama of Abortion: A Global Search for Consensus* (originally published in Portuguese in 2004 and published in Spanish in 2005).

José Barzelatto graduated from medical school at the University of Chile in December 1949 and completed postgraduate training in endocrinology and nuclear medicine at the Massachusetts General Hospital in Boston. At the University of Chile, he conducted research in endemic goiter, headed a clinical radioisotope laboratory that trained Latin American physicians, and was appointed associate professor of medicine. He was also a member of the Chilean Atomic Energy Commission, editor of the *Chilean Medical Journal,* and founder of the Chilean National Council for Research in Science and Technology.

From 1968 to 1975, he served as special advisor to the Organization of American States (OAS) Multilateral Program for the Development of Science and Technology in Washington, D.C. (a program that he helped establish).

From 1975 to 1989, he worked for the World Health Organization (WHO) in Geneva, Switzerland. For the last five years he served as director of the United Nations (UNDP/WHO/World Bank) Special Programme for Research and Training in Human Reproduction, a global effort supporting the development of fertility regulation methods (including epidemiological assessments of their efficacy and safety, social science research on human reproduction, and the development of research institutions in developing countries).

From 1989 to 1996, he was director of the Reproductive Health and Population Program of the Ford Foundation in New York, a program that contributed to the global conceptual shift from fertility reduction through the promotion of contraception to a more holistic vision centered on sexual and reproductive health and rights, education, and socioeconomic development.

From 1997 until 2006, the late José Barzelatto was vice president of the Center for Health and Social Policy (CHSP), a nongovernmental organization with international ventures aimed at improving social justice and health. He was also a member of the boards of CHANGE (Center for Health and Gender Equity) and IPPF/WH (International Planned Parenthood Federation, Western Hemisphere).